SpringerBriefs in Sociology

MW00780569

Series Editor

Robert J. Johnson
Department of Sociology, University of Miami, Miami, FL, USA

For further volumes:
http://www.springer.com/series/10410

Sherry Hamby · John Grych

The Web of Violence

Exploring Connections Among Different
Forms of Interpersonal Violence and Abuse

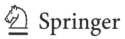 Springer

Sherry Hamby
Sewanee, The University of the South
Sewanee, TN
USA

John Grych
Department of Psychology
Marquette University
Milwaukee, WI
USA

ISSN 2212-6368
ISBN 978-94-007-5595-6
DOI 10.1007/978-94-007-5596-3
Springer Dordrecht Heidelberg New York London

ISSN 2212-6376   (electronic)
ISBN 978-94-007-5596-3   (eBook)

Library of Congress Control Number: 2012949126

Printed on acid-free paper

Springer is part of Springer Science+Business Media (www.springer.com)

Acknowledgments

One of the great pleasures of completing a project like this is the opportunity to reflect on all of those who have helped and supported us in our work.

We would like to thank Kaki Nix for her assistance with the literature review and Bridget Dolan for her assistance in preparing the bibliography. At Springer Publishing, we would like to thank our editor, Myriam Poort, for her initial interest and ongoing support. Also, we would like to acknowledge her senior assistant, Miranda Dijksman, for her always prompt and courteous communications throughout the process. Thanks also go to the production editor, Rangarajan Mathivanan, for supervising the creation of the cover and shepherding our manuscript into book form and also to Sundari for overseeing the creation of the proofs. We are also grateful to Robert J. Johnson, the editor of the SpringerBriefs Series in Sociology, for his constructive feedback that helped strengthen the final product. We would also like to offer our appreciation to the two reviewers for their comments on an earlier draft of the manuscript. We would like to thank Peter Van der Linden for introducing us to Myriam Poort.

Several of our colleagues are owed a debt of thanks for encouraging our thinking on the interconnections among forms of violence that are the focus of *Web of Violence*. Sherry would particularly like to thank David Finkelhor for first encouraging and supporting her to conduct integrative research beyond the silo of family violence and Heather Turner for many thought-provoking discussions on polyvictimization and related topics. John would like to express his gratitude to Ernie Jouriles and Jennie Noll for many stimulating and expansive discussions about this topic and many others. We would also like to thank Robert Geffner and Jacquelyn White, co-chairs of the National Partnership to End Interpersonal Violence, for creating a forum where we first jointly discussed many of the topics addressed in this book.

Over the years a number of other people have helped us to sustain this sometimes-challenging work and to stretch and stimulate our thinking. Some to whom we are especially grateful are David Jack Bell, Greg Fosco, Bernadette Gray-Little, Pat Kerig, Kristen Kracke, Kristin Lindahl, Neena Malik, Molly McCaffrey, and Tammy Russell. We would like to express our appreciation to the Departments of Psychology at Sewanee, the University of the South and Marquette University for support both tangible and intangible.

Many individuals—too many to count—who we have encountered through our clinical work, in the classroom, or in our broader social networks, have also contributed to our growing recognition of the interconnections among forms of violence. It is our hope that we will in some small way contribute to reducing poly-victimization and poly-perpetration of all types.

Finally, we are most grateful to our families for all that they do to support and encourage us in our work and in so much else. Al Bardi, Lynnaya Bardi Hamby, Julian Hamby Bardi, Janet Arnold-Grych, Alec Arnold Grych, and Aaron Arnold Grych have above all helped us to envision a world where fewer people's lives are touched by violence.

Contents

1   **The Case for Studying Co-occurrence** 1
The Cost of Compartmentalization 1
What is Gained by Focusing on Co-occurrence? 2
Benefits for Research 2
Benefits for Practice and Policy 4
Are There Costs to the Co-occurrence Approach? 4
Interconnections, Not Inevitabilities 6
The Plan of the Book 7
References 7

2   **Tracing the Threads of the Web: The Epidemiology
of Interconnections Among Forms of Violence and Victimization** 9
The Language of Co-occurrence 10
Gaps in Knowledge on Co-occurrence 11
Patterns Across Different Types of Violence 12
Poly-victimization: Co-occurrence Among Forms of
    Victimization 12
Poly-perpetration: Co-occurrence Among Forms of Perpetration 13
Dual Involvement in Violence as Both Perpetrator and Victim 14
Patterns Over Time 15
Revictimization: Ongoing Patterns of Victimization 16
Reperpetration: Ongoing Patterns of Offending 16
The Link Between Childhood Victimization and Adult
    Perpetration 17
Particularly Strong Linkages Between Forms of Violence 18
Gender and Co-occurrence 21
Gender Patterns for Single Forms of Violence 21
Gender and Co-occurrence: The Big Picture 24
Conclusions 24
References 25

3   The Causes of Interconnection.   29
  Conceptualizing the Causes of Interpersonal Violence   30
  Individual Factors   34
  Cognitive Processes.   34
  Emotional Processes   38
  Self-Regulation   40
  Personality.   40
  Biological Factors   41
  Situational Factors.   42
  The Behavior of Others.   43
  The Relationship Context   44
  Conclusion.   45
  References.   46

4   A Developmental Perspective on Interconnection   51
  The Developmental Course of Aggression   51
  The Development of Risk Factors for Violence   52
  Relationship with Caregivers   53
  Child Maltreatment   54
  Family Conflict and Exposure to Other Forms of Aggression   55
  Peer Relationships.   56
  Links Between Family and Peer Contexts.   58
  Romantic Relationships in Adolescence   59
  Links Among Peer, Dating, and Family Relationships   61
  Conclusion.   62
  References.   63

**5   Implications for Research: Toward a More Comprehensive
     Understanding of Interpersonal Violence**.   67
  Developing Models of Interconnection for Interpersonal
       Violence   67
  The Roles of Common and Specific Factors.   69
  Increase the Developmental Focus of Research   70
  Attend More to the Linkages Between Victimization
       and Perpetration   70
  Design Methods to Advance the Science of Co-occurrence   71
  Sampling   71
  Design Issues.   72
  Measurement.   73
  Improving Distinctions Between Limited and Severe
       Violence   74
  Data Analysis.   75
  Conclusion.   77
  References.   77

6 Implications for Prevention and Intervention: A More
   Person-Centered Approach 81
   Prevention 81
       How Compartmentalization Affects Prevention. 81
       Improving Prevention Through Greater Emphasis on
           Co-occurrence 82
       Next Steps: Advancing Prevention Through Explicit
           Emphasis on Co-occurrence. 83
       Challenges in Making Prevention More Informed by
           Co-occurrence 87
   Assessment 89
       How Compartmentalization Affects Assessment 89
       Improving Assessment Through Greater Emphasis on
           Co-occurrence 90
       Next Steps: Advancing Assessment Through Greater Emphasis
           on Co-occurrence 91
   Intervention 92
       How Compartmentalization Affects Intervention 92
       Next Steps: Advancing Intervention Through Greater
           Emphasis on Co-Occurrence 92
       Challenges in Making Assessment and Intervention More
           Informed by Co-occurrence 93
       Existing Efforts to Improve Intervention Through Greater
           Emphasis on Co-Occurrence 95
   Community-Level Interventions: Policy, Law, and Community
       Action. 97
       How Compartmentalization Affects Community-Level
           Interventions. 97
       Improving Community Approaches Through Greater
           Emphasis on Co-occurrence. 97
       Next Steps: Advancing Community Approaches Through
           Explicit Emphasis on Co-occurrence 98
       Challenges in Making Community-Level Approaches
           More Informed by Co-occurrence 99
   Conclusion. 100
   References. 100

7 Conclusion: Toppling the Silos. 105
   Extend and Expand Theory and Research. 106
   Integrate and Coordinate Prevention and Intervention Services 106
   Communicate and Collaborate 106
   Incentivize and Institutionalize 106
       Final Thoughts 107
   References. 108

Chapter 1
The Case for Studying Co-occurrence

The Cost of Compartmentalization

For decades, research examining different forms of interpersonal violence has proceeded in relative isolation. Large literatures have been generated on child maltreatment, bullying, intimate partner violence, teen dating violence, sexual violence, and elder abuse with few systematic efforts to understand connections among them. There are exceptions, such as work investigating links between intimate partner violence and child physical abuse, but for the most part, each field of study has developed its own conceptual models, knowledge base, and approaches to intervention. There are historical reasons that these "silos" have developed; different forms of violence have come to public and scientific attention at different times, and the initial work on each understandably sought to document the nature and extent of the problem and to identify ways to prevent it or aid its victims. Although much has been learned about each type of violence, the propensity for research, services, and even entire institutions to organize around single forms of violence or a few closely related types has significant costs as well.

By focusing in on particular types of violence, the field as a whole has failed to recognize the extent to which different forms of interpersonal violence are connected across contexts, over the lifespan from birth through adulthood, and in the lives of victims, perpetrators, and those involved in violence as both victim and perpetrator. Disciplinary silos slow the advance of scientific progress by restricting the flow of information about the causes and correlates of different forms of violence, resulting in the repeated reinvention of conceptual and methodological wheels and reduced opportunities for researchers in one subfield to learn from the insights gleaned in others. Studying the interconnections of different violence types can lead to more comprehensive understanding of how and why violence occurs and to more effective approaches to reducing the number of children, women, and men who become victims.

There have been studies documenting co-occurrence of different forms of violence in a surprisingly large number of disciplines of violence scholarship and

S. Hamby and J. Grych, *The Web of Violence*, SpringerBriefs in Sociology, DOI: 10.1007/978-94-007-5596-3_1, © The Author(s) 2013

practice, but most have addressed only two fairly specific forms of violence, and disciplinary silos and hyper-specialization have meant that this scholarship generally has been conducted in isolation from other work on co-occurrence. Although there have been calls to focus more on the relations among forms of violence in the past (Slep and Heyman 2001), only recently have there been concerted efforts to systematically assess the extent of interconnection across multiple forms of violence (e.g., Finkelhor et al. 2009). This work indicates that the overlap among different forms of violence, even seemingly diverse and unrelated forms, is so great that it can be difficult to identify a group of individuals who have sustained or perpetrated only a single form of violence (see Chap. 2). The high level of violence co-occurrence has important implications for research, intervention, and public policy, and the purpose of this book is to address how knowledge generated in multiple domains can be organized into a larger framework that illuminates the commonalities and patterns among them. We believe that greater recognition of these connections will lead to a more contextualized and comprehensive approach to research, prevention, and intervention on all forms of violence.

What is Gained by Focusing on Co-occurrence?

The most fundamental advantage of a co-occurrence perspective is that it more closely corresponds to the reality of many, if not most, people who are involved in violence in some way. Individuals do not carve up their experiences according to the disciplinary and subdisciplinary boundaries established by scientists, clinicians, and policymakers. Narrow labels misrepresent and minimize the true burden of violence. Awareness of the interconnections among different forms of violence will provide a more accurate understanding of how violence affects people's lives, which in turn will facilitate efforts to reduce violence and the suffering that it causes. In the next section, we briefly address the advantages of recognizing the interconnected nature of different forms of interpersonal violence for research and for practice.

Benefits for Research

More valid inferences. Studies of a particular type of violence typically identify victims on the basis of their experience with that type of violence, and infer that it is that type of victimization that is related to whatever outcomes are being studied. Any victim group, however, will include many individuals who have experienced victimization in several different domains at the hands of several different perpetrators. Consequently, although outcomes are typically attributed to the form of victimization that is the focus of the study, they are likely to be the result of multiple forms. The same issues hold for studies of perpetrators; single labels such as "batterer," "bully," or "rapist" will be incomplete depictions of many individuals' involvement in violence. Given the high degree of co-occurrence of all forms of violence, studies that assess only a single type of violence and then label the group with that form are fundamentally inaccurate.

Even more disconcertingly, many participants in the comparison group are also likely to be victims of some type of violence and may have many characteristics in common with the "victim" group. Finding minimal differences between "victims" and "nonvictims," or between "perpetrators" and "nonperpetrators," can lead to the conclusion that the particular form of violence has little or no effect on whatever construct is the focus of the study. This conclusion could be erroneous if the ostensibly nonviolent group included individuals who had experienced forms of violence that were not assessed in the study but share many of the same risk factors and consequences as the form that was the focus of the study.

More sophisticated etiological models. Even a cursory scan of the major violence disciplines will reveal tremendous overlap in the constructs hypothesized to act as risk factors and causal processes. For example, growing up in a violent home is one of the best-supported etiological factors for both perpetration and victimization of violence across contexts. Some behaviors, such as substance abuse, put people at risk for everything ranging from becoming a victim of sexual assault to perpetrating property crimes. Although much has been learned about violence through the isolated study of these risk factors, decades of research now suggest that the main risk factors can be grouped into a few categories (see Chap. 3). A more integrated framework can provide additional insights into the magnitude of the associations between particular risk factors and particular types of violence, and would have direct implications for practice by identifying which malleable risk factors should be specifically targeted in prevention and intervention programs to produce the largest impact.

A co-occurrence framework is also best suited for distinguishing factors that may be unique to particular types of interpersonal violence from risk factors common to all forms of violence. Indeed, it is not possible to identify unique risk factors without an appreciation for the commonalities across forms of violence. In some cases, there might also be unique aspects to more general factors. For example, communication and negotiation skills have been identified as important for avoiding several forms of violence (as both victim and perpetrator), but specific skills, such as negotiating birth control use, might be important for avoiding some kinds of sexual aggression or reproductive coercion. More detail on this is presented in Chap. 3.

More developmentally sensitive understanding of violence. Surprisingly, little attention has been given to the developmental context of many violence types. In many research studies and prevention programs, developmental context is implied simply by the targeted age range. Many bullying prevention programs are designed for middle school youth, for example, even though data do not suggest that the onset of bullying occurs in middle school. As we discuss in Chap. 4, the roots of many forms of interpersonal aggression can be found in early childhood, where adverse experiences can increase children's subsequent vulnerability to victimization and risk for perpetration. Tracing the interplay over time among cognitive, emotional, and biological factors, family processes, peer interactions, and the connections between victimization and perpetration can shed light on the common and unique risk factors for violence.

Benefits for Practice and Policy

Increased programming efficiencies. New ideas are needed to maximize the benefits from our existing (or even shrinking) resources. Many prevention and intervention programs have emerged from specific violence silos and are offered without regard for what other services a person is receiving or has already received, and we cannot afford to continue to duplicate efforts across programs and settings. Fragmented and overlapping approaches to intervention also may create confusing or even conflicting messages. One of the greatest areas of promise of a co-occurrence perspective is better coordination of services across different forms of violence. More coordinated responses are beginning to take hold for intimate partner violence, maltreatment, and children's exposure to violence, such as coordinated community response teams and children's advocacy centers, which proactively establish communication and cooperation across agencies.

More holistic approaches to prevention and intervention. Clinical intervention and prevention approaches often have a narrow focus, instead of more comprehensive, holistic, and person-centered approaches to issues of safety, healthy conflict resolution, and positive social development. Rather than having a raft of prevention programs that target individual problems (bullying, dating violence), systematically addressing factors that give rise to involvement in multiple forms of violence could have more powerful and longlasting effects (see Chap. 6).

Are There Costs to the Co-occurrence Approach?

We recognize that a focus on co-occurrence may seem to have disadvantages, especially at first blush. First and foremost, it suggests that researchers and practitioners must acquire expertise in forms of violence with which they may have only passing familiarity. For researchers, it is challenging enough to stay abreast of the advances in one area, much less try to master the theories, the empirical literature, and methods of several. For providers and policy makers, attending to co-occurrence may seem to add more responsibilities to institutions and personnel that are already strained with overwork. People who work in service-oriented institutions are often faced with new initiatives that seem to do little more than increase paperwork or require revamping of existing practices, sometimes with few apparent benefits.

As we will describe, adopting a co-occurrence perspective is not as daunting as it may seem, and we believe that any apparent disadvantages are far outweighed by the advantages. Managing the flood of new research and new practice innovations is a challenge; there has been much faster growth in knowledge generation than in the equally important tasks of knowledge synthesis and dissemination. New means of communication and integration are needed to meet this challenge, and the *Web of Violence* is intended to contribute to this process by serving as a concise overview of the conceptual and empirical work that form a basis for understanding the interconnections across forms of violence throughout the lifespan.

Fig. 1.1 Nested professional identities of violence researchers

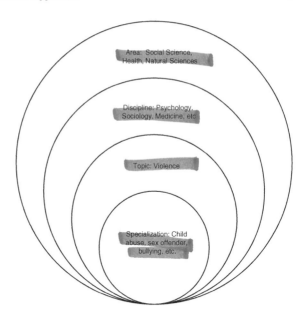

Area: Social Science, Health, Natural Sciences

Discipline: Psychology, Sociology, Medicine, etc

Topic: Violence

Specialization: Child abuse, sex offender, bullying, etc.

The co-occurrence framework can serve as scaffolding to help better organize existing knowledge and identify points of intervention. As will be seen in later chapters, there is enough overlap across silos that much of the theory and research is also likely to be already familiar to those who work in different fields. However, we also believe that acknowledging potential barriers is important, and briefly offer a few thoughts on questions that might be raised by the prospect of giving greater prominence to co-occurrence in future research and practice on violence.

Identity. Many professionals' identities are closely tied to their area of specialization, and we recognize that an increased focus on co-occurrence might require a shift in perspective for some. We have found it useful to think of professional identities in much the way that other social identities are constructed. Most people have multiple identities, such as researcher and parent, and multiple professional identities, such as researcher and teacher. Some identities can be thought of as nested, such as Floridian and American. We are not suggesting that people give up their identities as child abuse researchers or sex offender therapists, but rather to also view themselves as part of a larger community of violence professionals (see Fig. 1.1). There is the still broader context of disciplinary identities such as psychologist, sociologist, physician, or social worker. Because training and work roles are often organized around these identities, there is often more identification with the broader discipline than there is with one's own topic area.

Re-thinking past work. Another concern we have heard expressed is the implications for contemporary evaluations of past scholarship. Although we are sympathetic to the desire to hold past scholarship, perhaps especially one's own past work, in esteem, past work is probably best recognized for its role in the ongoing accumulation of knowledge. A continual process of change and improvement is an essential, if not the defining, characteristic of science; indeed, the more quickly that past work becomes obviously dated, the healthier perhaps the scientific enterprise is. The groundbreaking work in different subfields of violence in the 1960s, 1970s, and 1980s accomplished much to identify violence as a major social problem, including grossly under-recognized areas such as family violence and acquaintance rape. Early research also established the viability of empirical and quantitative approaches to studying crime and violence, including the then-surprising revelation that it was possible to learn much about violence through the method of self-report. Many of the institutions and laws in existence today can be directly traced to the increased social awareness created by this seminal research.

Nonetheless, the incredible value of these research efforts does not imply that 40-year-old methods are the best that can be developed, or that there is not still much we need to understand about virtually every form of violence. In this regard, we believe that the focus on co-occurrence not only highlights a greatly under-studied aspect of violent phenomena, but can also serve as a reminder that the scientific process is always a future-oriented endeavor that is focused on the novel: novel findings, novel methods, and novel research questions. There is increasing evidence of a new emphasis on synthesis and theoretical integration in research on violence, and we have endeavored to contribute to that process in our own work (Hamby 2005; Noll and Grych 2011). After many decades of fairly small-scale theoretical models focusing on one type of process, a second wave of violence scholarship is beginning to emerge that has started the task of exploring how mechanisms intersect, deepening our understanding of violence (Hamby 2011).

"That's not our mandate." We are sympathetic to the problems of chronic understaffing and high caseloads at many institutions that provide direct services. We also recognize that some providers, such as obstetricians or teachers, may not view their work as being related to violence at all. We are aware that one way to manage unrealistic workloads is to define an institution's responsibilities in narrow terms. Although no single clinician, caseworker, or advocate can single handedly change these realities, we believe that a more coordinated, comprehensive, and ultimately more holistic and person-centered approach will both better meet the public's needs and reduce some of the frustrations and stresses of front-line work with those who have sustained or perpetrated violence. The organizational structure of our social and human services has emerged largely through historical accident, as new needs were recognized. Although a large task, we believe some restructuring of services is warranted. Keeping people safe should be one of, if not the, primary mandate of our social and human services. This mandate should not be executed as though only certain kinds of safety seem to apply.

Interconnections, Not Inevitabilities

Finally, we want to note that even though we are focusing on the high rates of co-occurrence among diverse forms of offending and victimization, it should never be assumed that a person presenting with one form of victimization or perpetration always has experienced some other form, or that these associations are invariant over time. This is especially important when working with individuals or families in clinical or criminal justice settings. The variability in these patterns also becomes more notable when focusing on more specific forms of violence. For example, even though exposure to partner violence and child maltreatment are very closely related, not all children who are exposed to partner violence are maltreated, and not all maltreated children are exposed to partner violence.

The Plan of the Book ✳

In the following chapters, we describe the extent of the interrelationships among different forms of interpersonal violence, examine causal models that may explain these connections, and consider developmental processes that give rise to multiple forms of violence. Then, we will address in more detail what the research on co-occurrence means for future empirical investigations and for preventing and intervening with victims and perpetrators of violence. Finally, we conclude with a few comments on key issues and next steps. Each chapter was a collaborative effort and the final product equally reflects our thinking on the issues presented herein.

References

Finkelhor, D., Turner, H., Ormrod, R., & Hamby, S. (2009). Violence, abuse and crime exposure in a national sample of children and youth. *Pediatrics, 124*, 1411–1423.

Hamby, S. (2005). Measuring gender differences in partner violence: Implications from research on other forms of violent and socially undesirable behavior. *Sex Roles-Special Issue: Understanding Gender and Intimate Partner Violence, 52*(11/12), 725–742.

Hamby, S. (2011). The second wave of violence scholarship: Integrating and broadening theories of violence. *Psychology of Violence, 1*(3), 163–165.

Noll, J. G., & Grych, J. H. (2011). Read–react–respond: An integrative model for understanding sexual revictimization. *Psychology of Violence, 1*(3), 202–215.

Slep, A. S., & Heyman, R. (2001). Where do we go from here? Moving toward an integrated approach to family violence. *Aggression and Violent Behavior, 6*, 353–356.

The Plan of the Book

Chapter 2
Tracing the Threads of the Web: The Epidemiology of Interconnections Among Forms of Violence and Victimization

Interconnections among types of violence are embodied in such well-known concepts as the "intergenerational transmission of violence" (Ehrensaft et al. 2003) and "criminal careers" (Blumstein et al. 1988). Some specific linkages have been the focus of considerable attention. For example, in psychology, the "spillover" of aggression from interparental to parent–child relationships has been well documented (Appel and Holden 1998), and in criminology, there long has been interest in identifying criminal "specialists" versus criminal "generalists" who commit multiple types of crimes (e.g., Wijkman et al. 2011). Diverse forms of violence are, however, even more closely linked than suggested by these lines of inquiry. The latest research shows that virtually all types of violence are interrelated, even seemingly quite different types such as child maltreatment and robbery (e.g., Finkelhor et al. 2009). Rather than a linear chain of transmission or a single link, these interrelationships radiate out in multiple directions; they connect across different forms of violence, endure throughout individual life spans, and extend even over generations. The primary purpose of this chapter is to delineate the various types of overlap that exist and to describe the known extent of the overlap, or co-occurrence, among forms of violence. We employ the term "violence" broadly to refer to a wide range of intentionally perpetrated harms. We include the major types that have been the focus of scholarly and institutional attention: conventional crimes such as assault and robbery, child maltreatment, intimate partner violence (IPV), sexual offenses, bullying and other forms of peer violence, and exposure to violence through witnessing violence in the community or in the home. In addition to more accurately documenting the nature of interpersonal violence, describing variation in the strength of particular connections is important for understanding etiology and developmental trajectories, and so we identify some of the stronger linkages that have so far been identified.

Table 2.1 A co-occurrence framework for violence that integrates previous terminologies

Role: Involvement in violence		
Victim	Perpetrator	Both
	Single episode or emphasis on single type	
Mono-victim	*Mono-perpetrator*	*Mono-perpetrator–victim*
Also studied under the name of:		
Acute	Specialists	Bully victim
Isolated		Mutual IPV
Single form exposed		
	Multiplicity: Patterns across types of violence	
Poly-victim	*Poly-perpetrator*	*Poly-perpetrator–victim*
Also studied under the name of:		
Multiple type victim	Generalists	Delinquent victim
Multiple victim	Violent polymorphism	
Multiple crime-type victim		
Multiple form exposed		
Complex trauma		
	Repetitiveness: Patterns across time	
Repeat victim	*Repeat perpetrator*	*Repeat perpetrator–victim*
Also studied under the name of:		
Repeat victim	Recidivist	Cycle of violence
Chronic	Habitual offender	Intergenerational transmission
Complex trauma	Reconviction	
	Revolving doors	
	Career criminal	

The Language of Co-occurrence

As noted above, many different terms have evolved to describe different types of co-occurrence. Some are fairly specific, such as "bully-victim" and "mutual IPV", whereas others are broader, such as "habitual offender" or "career criminal" (See Table 2.1 for other examples). The terms used to represent particular associations are used almost exclusively by professionals in one discipline and consequently tend to promote compartmentalization rather than integration. Creating a common, internally consistent set of terms could serve to identify similar phenomena in different fields and facilitate communication across disciplines, but as far as we are aware, there have been no comprehensive efforts to create a systematic set of terms that could be used for all types of violence. In Table 2.1 we offer such a scheme; it utilizes different prefixes to designate multiple patterns of co-occurrence that can be used to describe victimization as well as perpetration, for adults as well as children, and across major forms of violence as well as across the lifespan.

First, we use the prefix "poly" to refer to the co-occurrence of different forms of violence. Thus, "polyvictimization," a term first introduced by David Finkelhor, Heather Turner, and Dick Ormrod (2007), describes multiple types of victimization (such as peer victimization and caregiver abuse). "Polyperpetration" involves committing multiple types of offenses (such as violence and property crime). We use "re" or "repeat" for the occurrence of the same type of violence over time. "Re-victimization" refers to repeated experiencing of one victimization type (such as multiple incidents of physical abuse) and "re-perpetration," correspondingly, refers to repeated commission of one type of violence (such as multiple rapes). Single episodes can be more precisely specified by using the prefix "mono," as in "mono-victimization" and "mono-perpetration." Finally, we will adopt the term "perpetrator–victim" to refer to anyone who has been involved in violence in both roles, so this will include bully victims, delinquent victims, and mutual IPV, but will also include other combinations of perpetration and victimization in the life of a single individual.

Gaps in Knowledge on Co-occurrence

Despite the long history of the study of some forms of co-occurrence, many gaps remain and violence scholarship has not yet fully integrated some of the key insights. We highlighted some of the advantages of a co-occurrence model in Chap. 1, including a shift to recognizing that co-occurrence is the norm, not the exception, and the importance of developing an overarching framework to incorporate findings on diverse interrelationships. There are two main gaps in our understanding of co-occurrence. The first is misconceptions created by the fairly accidental way the study of co-occurrence has developed. For example, there has been a great deal of attention paid to the overlap of morphologically similar victimizations, even though the form of violence has not been established as a key source of linkages. For example, there has been a great deal of study on the overlap between child abuse and exposure to interparental domestic violence, but almost all of this has focused on one form of abuse, child physical abuse. National Survey of Children's Exposure to Violence (NatSCEV) data indicate, however, that exposure to domestic violence is more closely linked to neglect and even sexual abuse than it is to physical abuse (Hamby et al. 2010). Similarly, NatSCEV data also indicate that although a past history of sexual victimization is associated with revictimization risk, other types of victimization also increase the risk of later sexual victimization (Finkelhor et al. 2011). The second gap, related to the first, is inattention to strong linkages across different forms of violence that do not "match." For example, the link between physical assault and sexual assault is very strong (Finkelhor et al. 2009), but has received relatively little study.

Finally, despite the growing body of the literature on co-occurrence, there continues to be an incident-specific focus in many violence professions, perhaps especially law enforcement and health care. Although we take this up from an intervention perspective in Chap. 6, regarding epidemiology we note that isolated incidents are the exception, not the rule. Perpetrators do not randomly select their targets, but engage in a complicated calculus of desirability and accessibility of the target that leads to some people perpetrating far more than others, and some people experiencing victimization far more than others. These cycles can be specific to one relationship, such as student to student or parent to child, or they can be operate at higher-order levels such as neighborhoods or even countries. The study of the patterns themselves is common in research on some types of violence, such as criminal offending, and rare in others, such as IPV, where individuals involved in a single incident are often treated the same as those with chronic involvement. Bearing these limitations in mind, we now turn to an overview of the main patterns of co-occurrence.

Patterns Across Different Types of Violence

One form of co-occurrence happens when an individual is victimized in multiple ways by multiple perpetrators. For example, a child might be abused in the home, bullied at school, and witness violence in their neighborhood. Some perpetrators are involved in multiple forms of violence too, as when individuals bully their peers and abuse their dating partners. Although the literature on co-occurrence is now large enough to offer some informed insights, surprisingly, for many forms of violence, linkages among different violence types have received relatively little study. For example, comparatively little is known about the overlap among different forms of adult victimization. Even the latest data under represent the true extent of co-occurrence because as yet there has been no comprehensive study of both victimization and perpetration. The causal and developmental pathways that contribute to these patterns of interconnection will be discussed in Chaps. 3 and 4. Here, we present an overview of basic patterns.

Poly-victimization: Co-occurrence Among Forms of Victimization

The vulnerabilities that expose a person to greater risk for one type of violence, such as unsafe neighborhoods or dysfunctional families, also increase the risks for many other types. Thus, co-occurrence is common for many forms of victimization.

Youth. Two of the largest studies on co-occurrence have focused on the interconnections among forms of youth victimization. The National Survey of Children's Exposure to Violence (NatSCEV, Finkelhor et al. 2009) and its smaller precursor, the Developmental Victimization Survey (Finkelhor et al. 2005) are the largest US surveys devoted to youth victimization. They provide nationally representative data on numerous forms of youth victimization, including several forms of physical assault, sexual victimization, child maltreatment, and witnessing violence. They also include offenses, such as neglect and statutory rape, which are crimes only when perpetrated against minors.

Results from both surveys indicate that there is significant overlap across all major victimization categories, including physical assault, sexual victimization, maltreatment, property crime, and exposure to violence. In NatSCEV, the average age-adjusted odds ratio (OR) for these overlaps was 2.7 for victimization occurring within the past year and 2.8 for lifetime victimization experiences. The strongest link was between physical victimization and sexual victimization. The risk of sexual victimization was 620 % higher (OR 6.2) for youth who had sustained at least one physical assault. The weakest link was between indirect exposure to violence and physical victimization. Although still a significantly elevated risk, youth who had been exposed to violence by knowing a victim, seeing the consequences (such as household burglary), or being told about an incident, without directly witnessing violence, were 40 % more likely to be physically assaulted than nonexposed youth (OR 1.4). For most types of violence, though, the experience of sustaining one form of victimization is associated with a doubling or tripling of the risk of any other form of victimization (Finkelhor et al. 2009). The Adverse Childhood Experiences study (Felitti et al. 1998), which involves retrospective reporting by adults, also supports the premise that many forms of youth victimization regularly co-occur.

Adults. Only recently has attention turned to the interrelationships among types of adult victimization. As outlined in more detail below, it is well known that some perpetrators commit more than one type of offense against adult victims. Probably, the best known case is IPV, which typically involves both psychological and physical aggression, and not infrequently involves sexual aggression and stalking by the intimate partner as well (Krebs et al. 2011; Straus et al. 1996). The most recent data reveal that these interconnections even operate on a daily level; in one study, physical IPV was 64 times more likely on a day when psychological IPV had occurred (Sullivan et al. 2012). More generally, a nationally representative survey of Latino women found that nearly two-thirds (63 %) of victimized women reported more than one type of victimization (Cuevas et al. 2010), with a mixed pattern of polyvictimization and revictimization being the most commonly reported pattern (multiple victimization types in childhood and/or adulthood with at least one type experienced more than once). A study of female IPV victims found that most had experienced other types of adversities, with more than half (58 %) experiencing physical assault by another family member and 42 % experiencing sexual assault by a family member (Graham-Bermann et al. 2011). As can be seen from these examples, most co-occurrence research on adult victimization takes a lifespan perspective, and more research is needed to understand how patterns of co-occurrence change across the trajectory of adulthood.

Poly-perpetration: Co-occurrence Among Forms of Perpetration

The "careers" of both juvenile and adult criminals are often grouped into categories based on the co-occurrence across types of violence and over time. Among the general public, many informal references to criminals use mono-perpetrator terms such as "burglar," "murderer," or "rapist." But, especially for criminals whose careers are not limited to an adolescent delinquent period, poly-perpetration is very common. As the term implies, poly-perpetrators do not limit themselves to one type of perpetration, but commit, for example, both violent and property crimes, or both sexual and nonsexual offenses (Blokland and van Wijk 2008; Moffitt 1993).

The generalization of criminal behavior typically starts at a very young age. For example, in a Dutch study of teens arrested for a sexual offense, already more than one in four had also been arrested for a nonsexual offense. Within 10 years, nearly half had been arrested again for a nonsexual offense (Blokland and van Wijk 2008). Generalization of offending often implies persistence over time, as different types of offenses accumulate. Poly-perpetrators are a small proportion of the population but commit a high percentage of all crimes. For example, they comprised 7 % of one longitudinal study of a Philadelphia birth cohort, but those 7 % were responsible for 70 % of rape arrests (Tracy et al. 1990). Poly-perpetration is also common among women arrested for sexual offenses. More than a quarter (27 %) of sex offending women commit multiple nonsexual offenses as well, and more than half committed multiple sexual offenses (Wijkman et al. 2011).

Dual Involvement in Violence as Both Perpetrator and Victim

Early research on violence almost universally classified individuals as either "perpetrators" or "victims"—and seldom both. Over the last two decades, however, researchers have found that many individuals are ensnared in dangerous situations or dangerous relationships as both perpetrators and victims. This type of co-occurrence has been most frequently examined in the fields of delinquency, bullying, and IPV (Lauritsen et al. 1991; Salmivalli and Nieminen 2002; Whitaker et al. 2007). Common terms to represent these interconnections include "delinquent-victims," "bully-victims," and, when a single dyad is involved, "mutual" or "reciprocal" violence, but we will apply the more general term of "perpetrator–victim."

This is a controversial area. Ideal victims receive more sympathy than flawed victims—and any hint of violent behavior can spoil the image of a victim (Loseke 1992). It can be especially challenging to avoid victim blaming when recognizing the interconnections between perpetration and victimization. Likewise, the image of victimized perpetrators can also be controversial, because it can be seen by some as a way of excusing violent behavior. We do not mean to imply victim blaming, or to avoid accountability for one's actions. Nonetheless, recognizing the interplay between victimization and perpetration is important for understanding violence and some studies suggest that perpetrator-victims are the largest group, larger than individuals who are predominantly perpetrators or predominantly victims (Cuevas et al. 2010). It also appears that perpetrator-victims may be at higher risk of injury than others (Whitaker et al. 2007). Methodologically, it is important

victim/offender overlap

to be careful about labeling individuals based on one or two reports of minor violence. The literature on youth delinquency and bullying (e.g., Cuevas et al. 2007; Salmivalli and Nieminen 2002) tends to be more sensitive to this than the IPV literature, where a person who pushes their partner once or twice in response to frequent violence and the partner who repeatedly engages in aggression would be categorized the same way. Nuances become apparent when more careful classifications are used. For example, children who are primarily victims may engage in limited acts of aggression, but these acts are much more likely to be reactive to others' aggression, versus the more proactive aggression of bully victims and primary bullies (Salmivalli and Nieminen 2002).

More recent research suggests there may even be meaningful subgroups within the group of delinquent victims (Cuevas et al. 2010). Some fit stereotypical images of youth involved in many violent activities and who have high victimization rates, with many incidents of perpetration and victimization involving peers. Others appear to be maltreated youth who act out in adolescence. And some victimized children do not engage in violent behavior, but do commit property crimes or other offenses (Cuevas et al. 2007).

In the field of IPV, such nuances are largely absent. "Mutuality" or reciprocity, in the IPV field, is often defined in all-or-none terms. For example, the following two scenarios would be treated equivalently. In the first couple, both spouses yell and swear when angry, and occasionally push or hit their partner. In another couple, one spouse frequently hits his (or her) partner when angry and after months or even years of this, the partner hits back. In most IPV research, both of these couples would be treated as equivalent members of the same class. We find it highly problematic to merely denote the presence of any perpetration without considering the patterning of the behavior over time (within interactions and over the course of many interactions). To do so misses the opportunities to identify important subgroups and variations based on frequency and severity, as has been done so fruitfully in research on bullying and delinquency. As we will discuss in more detail in Chap. 5, using the insights from subdisciplines of violence research to advance knowledge in other areas is an important positive benefit of the co-occurrence framework.

Patterns Over Time

Several longitudinal patterns have been identified. These include ongoing patterns of victimization, ongoing patterns of offending, and the link between childhood victimization and adult perpetration. The mechanisms thought to account for these patterns will be discussed in Chap. 4. Here, we will explore the strength of the associations over time. Patterns over time are not completely orthogonal to patterns across different types of violence, because except in war, riots, or other extreme circumstances, most poly-victimization and poly-perpetration will occur over a span of time. Still, research emphasizing patterns over time tends to emphasize different elements, especially longer time periods that often extend across developmental periods, such as childhood to adolescence or youth to adulthood.

It is important to note that none of these longitudinal patterns apply to the whole population or even the subset involved in a particular form of violence. Childhood experiences do not doom a person to an adulthood of violence and victimization. Nonetheless, as with other risks and vulnerabilities, the circumstances that led to an initial violence exposure can create conditions of ongoing risks, and rates of revictimization and offending are higher for people with early childhood exposures to violence.

Revictimization: Ongoing Patterns of Victimization

Revictimization most often refers to the repeated experience of a single form of victimization. Repeated sexual victimization, especially among females, has received the most attention (Noll and Grych 2011). Females who were sexually abused in childhood are two to three times more likely to be sexually assaulted in adulthood, compared to women with no childhood sexual abuse history (Barnes et al. 2009). In the National Intimate and Sexual Violence Survey (NISVS), more than a third (35 %) of women who had been raped in childhood were raped again in adulthood, versus an adult rape victimization rate of 14 % for women who were not raped as a child (Black et al. 2011). More generally, a childhood maltreatment history is associated with elevated risks for many adult victimizations, including physical assault, sexual assault, and stalking (Widom et al. 2008). These levels of revictimization only hint at true levels, though, because they focus on limited violence types.

Reperpetration: Ongoing Patterns of Offending

Criminal careers are also studied as developmental trajectories, where some individuals who are involved in delinquent acts at relatively young ages go on to become more serious offenders as adults. It has been noted that aggression is one of the most stable personality characteristics, rivaling even the stability of intelligence (Loeber and Stouthhamer-Loeber 1998). Aggressive behavior often emerges quite early and some children will be persistently aggressive throughout the span of childhood. These "life-course" repeat perpetrators account for the largest group of individuals who are violent in adulthood (Loeber and Stouthhamer-Loeber 1998).

Violent behavior does have an equally well-known age-related trajectory, however, in that almost everyone becomes less aggressive over time and the highest rate of serious offending occurs during late adolescence and young adulthood. Adolescence has been called a "self-limiting disease" (Vaillant 1977/1995, p. 159) because of this strong tendency to outgrow the worst violent and self-destructive behavior. The high stability coefficients are largely due to the fact that, although the absolute level of perpetration does decrease for the entire population over the span of development, the rank order of individuals tends to be highly stable. In other words, even though many highly aggressive individuals become less aggressive over time, they are still likely to be more aggressive than those who were consistently nonviolent from early childhood.

The Link Between Childhood Victimization and Adult Perpetration

People who have been hurt by violence might seem the least likely perpetrators of all. It has long been known, however, that this is not always so. Perhaps surprisingly, perpetrators are more likely to have a victimization history than the general population. Many victims do not go on to become offenders, however. There are also well-established gender differences in these patterns. Males comprise about 25–35 % of childhood sexual abuse victims, but make up about 95 % of sex offenders (Jonson-Reid and Way 2001). As with all of this literature, these patterns are indicative of elevated risks, not of certainties at the individual level.

Childhood Victimization History among Criminal Offenders. Given the markedly deviant behavior shown by many criminals, it is understandable that a great deal of attention has been given to the question of why and how their criminal behavior emerged. Across all population groups, childhood victimization rates are disturbingly high in most countries, but research indicates that childhood victimization is particularly elevated among those who are arrested for crime (Wijkman et al. 2011). One important, well-known caveat about this literature is the potential for self-serving reports: criminals may seek leniency or sympathy by reporting adverse childhood experiences. Nevertheless, some prospective research has also shown that maltreated children are more likely to be arrested as adults than nonmaltreated children (Widom and White 1997). In the US, several studies have found that the majority of sex offenders and juvenile delinquents report a childhood history of sexual or physical abuse. Reports of neglect and abuse are as high as 90 % (Leibowitz et al. 2011).

The Intergenerational Transmission of Family Violence. Although "intergenerational transmission" could refer to many longitudinal patterns, in practice this most often refers to childhood victims of maltreatment or exposure to family violence who go on to offend, as adults, against their own spouses and children. There has been some debate about the strength of this interconnection, motivated in part by concern that interconnections are often treated as inevitabilities not only by the general public, but also sometimes by providers and researchers (Widom 1989). It has often been noted that the strength of the association appears very different depending on the sampling frame. Among samples of batterers or child abusers, a majority often report abuse in their families of origin (e.g., Murphy et al. 1993). Yet this is a relatively small percentage of the population, and looked at from the other perspective—the number of maltreated or exposed children—only a minority go on to become perpetrators themselves (Widom 1989). Still, this is one of the strongest risk factors for perpetration. Sometimes the term "intergenerational transmission" also refers to the risk of being revictimized (see section on re-victimization). Taken together, these twin risks strongly indicate that early childhood exposure to violence leaves one vulnerable to multiple involvements with violence as an adult. More recent research suggests that exposure to interparental violence leaves one at risk of both later IPV perpetration and victimization, and that one's partner's exposure history also adds to this risk (Fritz et al. 2012).

Particularly Strong Linkages Between Forms of Violence

Existing evidence suggests that some forms of violence are more closely related than others. Understanding relative patterns of association is essential for untangling why co-occurrence happens, as particularly strong linkages may suggest similar etiologies. Unfortunately, what can be said about stronger and weaker linkages is limited by our current knowledge base, which has, as noted earlier in the chapter, tended to focus on interconnections among morphologically similar offenses. A few studies have, however, assessed the strengths of multiple patterns of interconnection and begin to shed light on which interconnections are stronger than others (e.g., Hamby et al. 2012). In Table 2.2, we present a selected set of associations between several forms of victimization. They include associations that have been frequently studied as well as connections between types of victimization that have received little attention and may be surprising to many. As the Table 2.2 shows, different forms of violence in the home are especially strongly linked. These and other patterns are discussed in more detail in the sections below, but one key point we would like to highlight here is that there are many strong connections that have received comparatively little study that could help shed further light on the mechanisms and interventions we will be addressing in later chapters. As can be seen in Table 2.2, even seemingly disparate forms of violence show some significant degree of interconnection in community samples. Understanding why some interconnections are stronger and some are weaker will be an important piece of advancing our understanding of co-occurrence and even of violence more generally.

Definitive conclusions about the magnitude of these associations are difficult to draw, however, because they may vary in different samples. For example, Appel and Holden (1998) found that IPV and physical child maltreatment were more strongly related in clinical samples consisting either of women from battered women's shelters or documented cases of abuse than in community samples. In general, problems of many types are likely to be more highly correlated in help seeking or law enforcement samples. Therefore, in order to provide a common reference point for the findings described below, we draw from studies utilizing community samples.

Child maltreatment and exposure to partner violence. Partner violence and child abuse share many common features, and it is not surprising that these phenomena often occur together (Bourassa 2007). Numerous studies indicate substantial overlap

Table 2.2 Examples of interconnections among forms of victimization in representative community samples

Interconnection	Strength of association (OR)
Well known, well-established interconnections	
Exposure to IPV and child physical abuse	5.0[a]
Exposure to IPV and teen dating violence victimization	3.8[a]
Physical IPV and stalking by intimate partner	7.0[d]
Physical IPV and sexual violence by intimate partner	2.4[d]
Strong but under-recognized interconnections	
Exposure to IPV and all other forms of maltreatment	
Psychological abuse	4.3[a]
Neglect	6.2[a]
Sexual abuse by known adult	5.2[a]
Custodial interference	9.2[a]
Any physical assault (by any perpetrator) and any sexual victimization	6.2[b]
Any witnessed violence and any sexual victimization	4.5[b]
Teen dating victimization and internet harassment	4.3[c]
Teen dating victimization and peer sexual harassment	5.3[c]
Weaker but still positive interconnections	
Exposure to IPV and peer relational aggression	1.7[a]
Exposure to IPV and exposure to community violence	2.1[a]
Any property crime and any sexual victimization	3.2[b]
Teen dating victimization and exposure to community violence	1.5[c]
Psychological IPV and physical violence by nonpartner	2.7[d]

Note OR = Odds ratio. The total number of possible interconnections is quite large and this table is not meant to be an exhaustive list. To date, most interconnections that have been studied have been found to be significantly positive. We focused on victimization because there are more nationally representative survey data available for victimization than perpetration (which is more often limited to official records or small convenience samples).
ORs for [a], [b], [c], and [d] have been adjusted to approximate the true relative risk (in the case of [d], that adjustment has been computed for this table). ORs for [a], [c], and [d] control for multiple demographics. ORs for [b] control for age.
[a]Hamby et al. (2010)
[b]Finkelhor et al. (2009)
[c]Hamby et al. (2012)
[d]Krebs et al. (2011)

lifetime overlap

between witnessing partner violence and child maltreatment (Appel and Holden 1998; Jouriles et al. 2008). In NatSCEV, the past year rate of physical abuse among children who had witnessed partner violence in the same year was 17.6 %. The lifetime overlap was even higher, with nearly a third (31 %) of children who had witnessed partner violence also experiencing physical abuse (Hamby et al. 2010).

Most research on the co-occurrence of exposure to partner violence and child abuse has focused on a single form of maltreatment, child physical abuse.

Although the shared physical assault component may make this seem a natural choice, the NatSCEV data show that all types of maltreatment are elevated among child witnesses to partner violence. Across multiple forms of maltreatment, youth who witness partner violence have rates of maltreatment that are 300–900 % higher than those for other youth (Hamby et al. 2010). Over the course of a lifetime, more than half (56.8 %) of youth IPV witnesses were also maltreated. Looking at some particular forms of maltreatment, fully 72 % of all youth who had ever experienced custodial interference had also witnessed partner violence. More than 60 % of neglect victims and more than 70 % of victims of sexual abuse by a known adult had also witnessed partner violence.

Teen dating violence. Teen dating violence provides an example of a form of violence that is almost always studied in isolation from other types of violence. Existing data, however, suggest that this focus does not accurately reflect reality. As with other forms of violence, teen dating violence is typically only one form of involvement in violence. Indeed, in the NatSCEV, every single youth who reported teen dating victimization also reported at least one other form of victimization. Within this general finding of polyvictimization, however, was also strong evidence for differences in the strength of the interconnections. In particular, many different forms of sexual victimization are very closely related to teen dating violence. The rate of teen dating violence among victims of rape was 25 %, or one in four, compared to 6.1 % for nonvictims, or approximately 1 in 16. Also notably, teen dating violence was particularly associated with some adult-perpetrated sexual offenses. The association with statutory rape was the highest for all forms of victimization, with fully half (50 %) of all youth in sexual relationships with much older partners (5 or more years older) also reporting teen dating violence. More than one in four youth (28.6 %) who had experienced an unwanted exposure by an adult also reported being a victim of teen dating violence (Hamby et al. 2012). Family violence was also especially closely associated with teen dating violence. More than half of teen dating violence victims have a history of some form of child maltreatment, with 44 % reporting physical abuse by a caregiver. More than two out of three youth had witnessed an assault between other family members. Other research also supports the link between exposure to family violence and teen dating violence (Jouriles et al. 2012).

Stronger links among forms of perpetration. As with victimization, some forms of perpetration are more closely related than others. Research suggests that poly-perpetrators who primarily commit violent and property crimes are more likely to commit rape versus sexual offenses such as child molestation and exhibitionism, which were more common among mono-perpetrators of sexual offenses (Blokland and van Wijk 2008). A study of female sex offenders similarly found that non-contact sexual offenses, such as taking illegal photos of minors, were perpetrated almost exclusively by mono or repeat perpetrators of sexual crimes and did not occur in the arrest histories of poly-perpetrating women who also committed violent or property crimes (Wijkman et al. 2011). Other researchers have also shown that sex offenders who target adult women are more likely to be poly-perpetrators than sex offenders who target children (Lussier 2005).

Gender and Co-occurrence

Determining whether these patterns are similar across key demographic subgroups is an important question not only for advancing a basic understanding of co-occurrence, but also for determining priorities for prevention and intervention. Gender has been studied more than any other sociodemographic characteristic, and is a topic of considerable debate in some disciplines. A co-occurrence approach to gender patterns in violence can inform these debates. Some services and institutions are also organized at least in part by gender, including shelters for battered women, batterers intervention programs, and jails, adding to the importance of accurately understanding how gender influences co-occurrence.

Gender Patterns for Single Forms of Violence

In some fields there is near-universal consensus on the existence of gender differences in violent behavior, whereas in others it is a hotly contested issue. In the former category include most conventional crimes. There is virtually universal agreement that men commit more homicides, sexual assaults, and robberies than women. Gang involvement is widely acknowledged to be more common among men. Homicide, robberies, and sexual offenses have a male-to-female perpetration ratio of approximately 9:1, whereas for nonlethal physical assault, the ratio is approximately 3 or 4:1 (for reviews, see Hamby 2005, 2009). Further, all types of measures (e.g., self-report, crime statistics) find these patterns consistently. In the US, for example, the large National Crime Victimization Survey (NCVS), consistently finds this pattern for victim self-report, as do official records such as the Uniform Crime Report and the National Incident-Based Reporting System, which tracks the public's reports to the police, regardless of whether they lead to an arrest. Similar data sets from other countries are consistent with these findings. The ratio of male-to-female perpetration is similar for major violent crime categories even though self-report surveys usually produce higher estimates than official statistics, presumably because not all offenses are reported to authorities.

On the other hand, there is considerable debate about other types of violence, such as IPV and bullying. We develop these examples in some detail to show how the co-occurrence framework can enhance our understanding of specific forms of violence as well.

IPV. Many researchers commonly assert that "most" data support the assertion that females perpetrate as much, if not more, physical IPV than males; however, this is true for only one particular methodology: self-report using perpetrator-specific behavioral checklists, such as the Conflict Tactics Scales (Straus et al. 1996) and the Conflict in Adolescent Dating Relationships Inventory (Wolfe et al. 2001). Other large, nationally representative, self-report surveys find more male than female perpetration, including the NISVS (NISVS; Black et al. 2011), the

MINOR VIOLENCE → MORE False Pos.

National Violence Against Women Survey (Tjaden and Thoennes 2000), and the NCVS. These data are consistent with reports to law enforcement, arrests, and homicide data, which also point to more male perpetration of IPV, although they do also all find evidence for some female perpetration. Furthermore, questions on witnessing violence between one's parents also show more male than female perpetration (Hamby et al. 2011a). Behavioral checklists could be more valid than all of these other methods, but as yet there are no data suggesting this.

The lack of consistency across measures is due to multiple factors (for more detailed reviews, see Hamby 2005, 2009). We highlight two here. First, much of the research using CTS-type checklists has been done with younger samples. Data from other methods, such as reports to law enforcement, show that boys and girls are more similar (although not equal) in rates of IPV perpetration than adult males and females (Snyder and McCurley 2008). Second, methods differ in the severity of violence that they are most sensitive to. Crime statistics tend to capture the more serious end of the violence continuum, whereas self-report questionnaires typically include many items assessing minor aggression. Measures that emphasize minor violence are more susceptible to false positives, which are behaviors that are physically forceful but do not meet the traditional definition of aggression (i.e., behavior intended to cause harm). These can include pushing, grabbing, and hitting that occurs while joking around, "wrestling," or even flirting, as well as other physical but mutually acceptable interactions. In most surveys, most self-reported violence is minor, and there is evidence that female perpetration rates are estimated with more false positives than males, because female perpetration is more often described as horseplay or joking around than male perpetration (e.g., Perry and Fromuth 2005). Further, this sort of physical horseplay is more typical of adolescents and young adults than older adults, making teen dating violence data even more difficult to interpret than adult IPV. False positives make it more challenging to distinguish "signal" from the "noise" in measures of violence, and no existing methodology accurately discriminates between acts that fall near the definitional borders of violence versus playful or other nonaggressive uses of physical force.

Overall, we are more confident in drawing conclusions from patterns that can be observed across multiple methodologies than those obtained by a single method. Applying this standard to existing data on physical IPV alone, the most scientifically defensible conclusions at this point are that: (a) males perpetrate more injurious violence than females; (b) gender differences are smaller for less violent forms of behavior; (c) rates of IPV are more similar for males and females in adolescence than in adulthood. More definitive conclusions about gender differences in the perpetration of milder forms of aggression must await more detailed and nuanced measurement of these types of violence.

The relationship between gender and violence becomes more clear when we broaden the focus from single forms of violence to interconnections between forms of violence. In the following sections, we show how greater attention to co-occurrence can further inform our understanding of gender and violence.

Co-occurrence and IPV. The seeming parity in male and female aggression is partly due to ignoring sexual violence between intimate partners. Sexual activity

significant impacts 191 % higher

is one of the key distinguishing features of intimate relationships, and assessments that omit violence in this important domain are inevitably incomplete. Men are much more likely to perpetrate both sexual and physical violence than are women, and so adult women are more likely to be IPV poly-victims than adult men.

In NISVS, the rate of co-occurring forms of IPV was only 8 % for adult male IPV victims, with almost all of that accounted for by men who experienced both physical violence and stalking. In contrast, more than a third (36 %) of female IPV victims reported sustaining more than one type of IPV victimization—a rate more than four times higher than the male rate of IPV poly-victimization. The most common pattern of co-occurrence for women was also physical violence and stalking, but more than a third (34.5 %) of the poly-victimized group had experienced all three types measured in that study, physical violence, stalking, and rape.

Co-occurrence has a marked impact on estimates of gender patterns. In NISVS (Black et al. 2011), physical IPV victimization was slightly higher for females, but not by a large margin: 28 % of men reported physical IPV victimization, versus 33 % of women. In other terms, physical IPV victimization was 16 % higher for women than men. If rape and stalking are included, however, the total prevalence rate was 25 % higher for women than men (36 % females; 29 % males). In another indicator that speaks to the false positive issue, if incidents were limited to those with significant psychological, physical, social, or work impacts, then the victimization rate for women was 191 % higher than it was for men (29 % of women vs. 10 % of men).

These patterns appear to be somewhat different for teen dating violence. Physical teen dating violence also highly co-occurs with many other forms of victimization, but these patterns of co-occurrence appear to be largely similar for boys and girls. Including sexual victimizations, however, does reduce seeming gender parity for teens as well, and focusing on incidents that were injurious or frightening eliminates it.

Bullying and other peer aggression. A focus on co-occurrence can also help illuminate other controversies in gender patterns for violence. It is commonly perceived that girls are more relationally aggressive than boys, although a recent meta analysis found no evidence for gender differences in peer relational aggression (Card et al. 2008). The co-occurrence of peer relational, verbal, and physical aggression is different for boys and girls, and this probably accounts for some common misperceptions about gender differences. Boys are much more likely to be poly-perpetrators of physical and relational aggression, including bullying through physical intimidation and harassment (taking lunch money, threatening, vandalizing lockers or belongings, etc.). Girls are more likely to be mono-perpetrators of just relational aggression (or mono-victims of relational aggression), which may contribute to the impression that the best exemplar of relational aggression is female behavior. A subset of girls also appear to follow a fairly gender-specific developmental trajectory, where their physical aggression decreases across the school years, as it does for most youth, but relational aggression increases (Coté et al. 2007). For boys, these two forms of aggression are more highly correlated.

These different patterns of co-occurrence combine with the different, gendered content of peer aggression. Boys often sexually harass other boys by impugning their sexuality or verbally harass peers by questioning their adherence to the "boy code," which involves living up to standards of emotional stoicism, personal honor, and enjoyment of physical force (Pollack 2006). Many measures of relational aggression, however, do not include items that assess these forms of aggression, and thus can give mistaken impressions of the peer climate for boys. Girls' relational aggression often focuses on relationships themselves—who is liked, who is not. Although girls' sexuality is often impugned too, girls are more typically expected to walk a narrow (if not nonexistent) line between being deemed too sexually naive or too sexually promiscuous. Of course, all of this content largely ignores the limited agency of adolescents or pre-adolescents to control or even understand these aspects of their behaviors or personality.

Gender and Co-occurrence: The Big Picture

The patterns noted in both of these specific examples extend more broadly. Males are more likely to be poly-perpetrators for acts ranging from criminal offending to school aggression. The patterns are more variable for victimization. Evidence suggests that boys are more often poly-victims than girls (Turner et al. 2010), largely because of higher rates of exposure to community violence and more experiences of peer physical assault. Among youth, male-on-male violence is the most common pattern for a wide variety of offenses (Hamby et al. 2011b), and the most common pattern of a great deal of criminal offending, including homicide, is also male on male. Thus, this creates higher levels of not only of poly-perpetration but also poly-victimization. For other types of victimization, such as IPV, women are more likely to be poly-victims than men (Black et al. 2011).

Males also typically have different developmental trajectories of co-occurrence than females. Males who are victimized in early childhood are more likely to have dual involvement in violence as perpetrator-victims, while females are more likely to be revictimized. Some females perpetrate high rates of relational aggression without physical aggression, while physical and relational aggression tends to stay more closely linked for boys (Coté et al. 2007). Of course, exceptions to every pattern exist. There are substantial numbers of female poly-perpetrators, female perpetrator victims, and male repeat victims. A better understanding of how co-occurrence varies by gender offers promise as one avenue for advancing our understanding of how men and women are involved in violence.

Conclusions

The existing epidemiology on co-occurrence among forms of violence indicates that extensive overlap is the norm, not the exception. Although many violence professionals are aware of particular linkages related to their area of specialty, there needs to be greater recognition that the web of violence extends over time, across the lifespan and even through generations. Interconnections extend across settings and relationships. Much existing research has focused on the interconnections of seemingly similar types of violence, such as the overlap between child physical abuse and exposure to domestic violence, or an individual who was physically abused as a child turning into a parent perpetrator. The latest data, however, suggest that these morphological similarities do not create stronger linkages than other interconnections. Rather, these interconnections occur because the causal antecedents and developmental trajectories are similar for many forms of violence and victimization. For example, all forms of family violence are closely interrelated—not just different types of physical family violence—because deficits in emotion regulation and other key causes of violence can create multiple problems in the family context and can be passed across family members via social learning or other mechanisms. In the Chap. 3, we synthesize existing knowledge on the etiology of the web of violence.

References

Appel, A., & Holden, G. (1998). The co-occurrence of spouse and physical child abuse: A review and appraisal. *Journal of Family Psychology, 12*(4), 578–599.

Barnes, J., Noll, J., Putnam, F. W., & Trickett, P. (2009). Sexual and physical revictimization among victims of severe childhood sexual abuse. *Child Abuse and Neglect, 33*(7), 412–420.

Black, M., Basile, K., Breiding, M., Smith, S., Walters, M., Merrick, M., et al. (2011). *The national intimate and sexual violence survey: 2010 summary report*. Atlanta: Centers for Disease Control and Prevention.

Blokland, A., & van Wijk, A. (2008). Criminal careers of Dutch adolescent sex offenders: A criminological perspective. In M. Smith (Ed.), *Child sexual abuse: Issues and challenges* (pp. 203–219). Hauppage: Nova Science Publishers, Inc.

Blumstein, A., Cohen, J., Das, S., & Moitra, S. (1988). Specialization and seriousness during adult criminal careers. *Journal of Quantitative Criminology, 4*(4), 303–345.

Bourassa, C. (2007). Co-occurrence of interparental violence and child physical abuse and it's effect on the adolescents' behavior. *Journal of Family Violence, 22*, 691–701.

Card, N., Stucky, B. D., Sawalani, G. M., & Little, T. D. (2008). Direct and indirect aggression during childhood and adolescence: A meta-analytic review of gender differences, intercorrelations, and relations to maladjustment. *Child Development, 79*(5), 1185–1229.

Coté, S., Vaillancourt, T., Barker, E., Nagin, D., & Tremblay, R. (2007). The joint development of physical and indirect aggression: Predictors of continuity and change during childhood. *Development and Psychopathology, 19*, 37–55.

Cuevas, C., Finkelhor, D., Turner, H., & Ormrod, R. (2007). Juvenile delinquency and victimization: A theoretical typology. *Journal of Interpersonal Violence, 22*(12), 1581–1602.

Cuevas, C., Sabina, C., & Picard, E. (2010). Interpersonal victimization patterns and psychopathology among Latino women: Results from the SALAS study. *Psychological Trauma: Theory, Research, Practice, and Policy, 2*(4), 296–306.

Ehrensaft, M., Cohen, P., Brown, J., Smailes, E., Chen, H., & Johnson, J. (2003). Intergenerational transmission of partner violence: A 20-year prospective study. *Journal of Consulting and Clinical Psychology, 71*(4), 741–753.

Felitti, V. J., Anda, R. F., Nordenberg, D., Williamson, D. F., Spitz, A. M., Edwards, V., et al. (1998). Relationship of childhood abuse and household dysfunction to many of the leading causes of death in adults. *American Journal of Preventive Medicine, 14*(4), 245–258.

Finkelhor, D., Turner, H., Ormrod, R., & Hamby, S. L. (2005). The victimization of children and youth: A comprehensive, national survey. *Child Maltreatment, 10*(1), 5–25.

Finkelhor, D., Ormrod, R., & Turner, H. (2007). Poly-victimization: A neglected component in child victimization. *Child Abuse and Neglect, 31*, 7–26.

Finkelhor, D., Turner, H., Ormrod, R., & Hamby, S. (2009). Violence, abuse and crime exposure in a national sample of children and youth. *Pediatrics, 124*, 1411–1423.

Finkelhor, D., Turner, H., Shattuck, A., & Hamby, S. (2011). The role of general victimization vulnerability in childhood sexual re-victimization. Durham, NH: Crimes Against Children Research Center.

Fritz, P. A. T., Slep, A. M. S., & O'Leary, K. D. (2012). Couple-level analysis of the relation between family-of-origin aggression and intimate partner violence. *Psychology of Violence, 2*(2), 139–153. doi:10.1037/a0027370.

Graham-Bermann, S., Sularz, A., & Howell, K. (2011). Additional adverse events among women exposed to intimate partner violence: Frequency and impact. *Psychology of Violence, 1*(2), 136–149.

Hamby, S. (2005). Measuring gender differences in partner violence: Implications from research on other forms of violent and socially undesirable behavior. *Sex Roles-Special Issue: Understanding Gender and Intimate Partner Violence, 52*(11/12), 725–742.

Hamby, S. (2009). The gender debate on intimate partner violence: Solutions and dead ends. *Psychological Trauma, 1*(1), 24–34.

Hamby, S., Finkelhor, D., Turner, H., & Ormrod, R. (2010). The overlap of witnessing partner violence with child maltreatment and other victimizations in a nationally representative survey of youth. *Child Abuse and Neglect, 34*, 734–741.

Hamby, S., Finkelhor, D., Turner, H., & Ormrod, R. (2011a). *Children's exposure to intimate partner violence and other family violence (NCJ232272)*. Washington: U.S. Department of Justice.

Hamby, S., Finkelhor, D., Turner, H., & Ormrod, R. (2011b). *Perpetrator & victim gender patterns for 21 forms of youth victimization in the National Survey of Children's Exposure to Violence*.

Hamby, S., Finkelhor, D., & Turner, H. (2012). Teen dating violence: Co-occurrence with other victimizations in the National Survey of Children's Exposure to Violence (NatSCEV). *Psychology of Violence, 2*(2), 111–124. doi:10.1037/a0027191.

Jonson-Reid, M., & Way, I. (2001). Adolescent sexual offenders: Incidence of childhood maltreatment, serious emotional disturbance, and prior offenses. *American Journal of Orthopsychiatry, 71*(1), 120–130.

Jouriles, E., McDonald, R., Slep, A., Heyman, R., & Garrido, E. (2008). Child abuse in the context of domestic violence: Prevalence, explanations, and practice implications. *Violence and Victims, 23*(2), 221–235.

Jouriles, E., Mueller, V., Rosenfield, D., McDonald, R., & Dodson, M. C. (2012). Teens' experiences of harsh parenting and exposure to severe intimate partner violence: Adding insult to injury in predicting teen dating violence. *Psychology of Violence, 2*(2), 125–138. doi:10.1037/a0027264.

Krebs, C., Breiding, M., Browne, A., & Warner, T. (2011). The associations between different types of intimate partner violence experienced by women. *Journal of Family Violence, 26*, 487–500.

Lauritsen, J. L., Sampson, R., & Laub, J. (1991). The link between offending and victimization among adolescents. *Criminology, 29*, 265–292.

Leibowitz, G., Laser, J., & Burton, D. (2011). Exploring the relationships between dissociation, victimization, and juvenile sexual offending. *Journal of Trauma and Dissociation, 12*(1), 38–52.

Loeber, R., & Stouthhamer-Loeber, M. (1998). Development of juvenile aggression and violence: Some common misconceptions and controversies. *American Psychologist, 53*(2), 242–259.

Loseke, D. R. (1992). *The battered woman and shelters: The social construction of wife abuse.* Albany: State University of New York Press.

Lussier, P. (2005). The criminal activity of sexual offenders in adulthood: Revisiting the specialization debate. *Sexual Abuse: A Journal of Research and Treatment, 17*(3), 269–292.

Moffitt, T. E. (1993). Adolescence-limited and life-course-persistent antisocial behavior: A developmental taxonomy. *Psychological Review, 100*(4), 674–701.

Murphy, C. M., Meyer, S., & O'Leary, K. D. (1993). Family of origin violence and MCMI-II psychopathology among partner assaultive men. *Violence and Victims, 8*, 165–176.

Noll, J. G., & Grych, J. H. (2011). Read–react–respond: An integrative model for understanding sexual revictimization. *Psychology of Violence, 1*(3), 202–215.

Perry, A., & Fromuth, M. E. (2005). Courtship violence using couple data: Characteristics and perceptions. *Journal of Interpersonal Violence, 20*(9), 1078–1095.

Pollack, W. S. (2006). The "war" *for* boys: Hearing "real boys" voices, healing their pain. *Professional Psychology: Research and Practice, 37*(2), 190–195.

Salmivalli, C., & Nieminen, E. (2002). Proactive and reactive aggression among school bullies, victims, and bully-victims. *Aggressive Behavior, 28*(1), 30–44.

Snyder, H. N., & McCurley, C. (2008). *Domestic assaults by juvenile offenders.* Washington: Office of Juvenile Justice & Delinquency Prevention.

Straus, M. A., Hamby, S., Boney-McCoy, S., & Sugarman, D. (1996). The revised conflict tactics scales (CTS2): Development and preliminary psychometric data. *Journal of Family Issues, 17*(3), 283–316.

Sullivan, T. P., McPartland, T. S., Armeli, S., Jaquier, V., & Tennen, H. (2012). Is it the exception or the rule? Daily co-occurrence of physical, sexual, and psychological partner violence in a 90-day study of substance-using, community women. *Psychology of Violence, 2*(2), 154–164. doi:10.1037/a0027106.

Tjaden, P., & Thoennes, N. (2000). *Extent, nature, and consequences of intimate partner violence: Findings from the national violence against women survey.* Washington: National Institutes of Justice.

Tracy, P. E., Wolfgang, M. E., & Figlio, R. (1990). *Delinquency careers in two birth cohorts.* New York: Plenum.

Turner, H., Finkelhor, D., & Ormrod, R. (2010). Poly-victimization in a national sample of children and youth. *American Journal of Preventive Medicine, 38*(3), 323–330.

Vaillant, G. E. (1977/1995). *Adaptation to life.* Cambridge, MA: Harvard University Press.

Whitaker, D., Haileyesus, T., Swahn, M., & Saltzman, L. (2007). Differences in frequency of violence and reported injury between relationships with reciprocal and nonreciprocal intimate partner violence. *American Journal of Public Health, 97*(5), 941–947.

Widom, C. (1989). Does violence beget violence? A critical examination of the literature. *Psychological Bulletin, 106*, 3–28.

Widom, C., & White, H. R. (1997). Problem behaviours in abused and neglected children grown up: Prevalence and co-occurrence of substance abuse, crime and violence. *Criminal Behavior and Mental Health, 7*, 287–310.

Widom, C., Czaja, S., & Dutton, M. A. (2008). Childhood victimization and lifetime revictimization. *Child Abuse and Neglect, 32*, 785–796.

Wijkman, M., Bijleveld, C., & Hendriks, J. (2011). Female sex offenders: Specialists, generalists and once-only offenders. *Journal of Sexual Aggression, 17*(1), 34–45.

Wolfe, D., Scott, K., Reitzel-Jaffe, D., Wekerle, C., Grasley, C., & Straatman, A. (2001). Development and validation of the conflict in adolescent dating relationships inventory. *Psychological Assessment, 13*(2), 277–293.

violence begets more violence
 (1 victim. leads to perpetration
 (2 victimization leads to re-vict
 (3 perpetration leads to re perp

Chapter 3
The Causes of Interconnection

vulnerability & risk

A wide range of conceptual models has been developed to explain the origins of various forms of interpersonal violence. Most focus on a single type of violence, but there is considerable consistency in the risk factors and etiological processes they describe. This consistency indicates that most poly-victimization and poly-perpetration emerges from similar conditions of vulnerability and risk, and suggests that one reason that different forms of violence co-occur is because they share common causal mechanisms (Fig 3.1). Perhaps the most prominent risk factor identified across diverse types of violence is prior exposure to violence; thus, a second source of interconnection is that many of the mechanisms hypothesized to give rise to violence are themselves sequelae of experiences with abuse, maltreatment, and aggression. In this chapter, we highlight common processes identified in etiological models of different forms of violence to illustrate how theoretical integration could advance understanding of violence that occurs in multiple contexts and relationships. Many of these processes also are important for explaining how violence can beget more violence, including victimization leading to perpetration, victimization to re-victimization, and perpetration to re-perpetration; in the next chapter, we will examine the developmental processes by which early experiences with violence can directly increase vulnerability to later perpetration and victimization.

Our focus on common factors does not imply that causal mechanisms unique to particular forms of violence do not exist; indeed, a comprehensive model of interpersonal violence needs to explain why one type of violence occurs rather than another, and common processes are insufficient for doing so. However, the heuristic framework that we describe below allows for specific as well as general effects and consequently can account for discontinuities as well as continuities across types of violence.

S. Hamby and J. Grych, *The Web of Violence*, SpringerBriefs in Sociology,
DOI: 10.1007/978-94-007-5596-3_3, © The Author(s) 2013

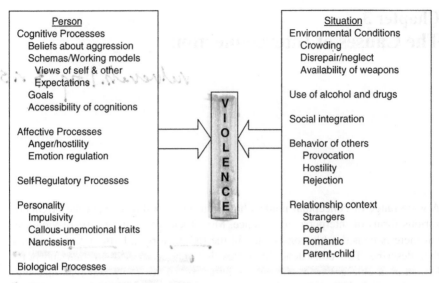

Fig. 3.1 Framework of etiological factors relevant to most forms of interpersonal violence

Conceptualizing the Causes of Interpersonal Violence

Most conceptual models developed for particular types of violence address perpetration or victimization, but not both. There also tends to be more overlap in the processes proposed to explain different forms of perpetration or different forms of victimization than there is for perpetration and victimization of the same violence type. Aggression is motivated, goal-driven behavior, and many of the intrapersonal characteristics that make some people more likely to engage in violence in one situation also would be expected to be present in other situations. In contrast, victimization often is a product of circumstances; individuals need not have any particular characteristics to be a target of aggression. However, conceptualizing perpetration primarily as a product of individual characteristics and victimization as a product of situational factors is overly simplistic. As we discuss below, situational factors play an important role in evoking aggressive behavior, and there are individual characteristics that make some individuals more vulnerable to victimization than others. In fact, many of the same classes of constructs included in models of perpetration also appear in models of victimization (e.g., biological stress response, substance use, poverty), suggesting that there may be shared etiological pathways for at least some forms of victimization and perpetration. Further, the line between perpetration and victimization is blurred when violence occurs in the midst of an interaction or ongoing relationship in which both partners engage in aggression at some point. Some individuals also are involved as both perpetrator and victim in larger group settings, such as schools or neighborhood gangs. Thus, factors usually linked specifically to victimization or to perpetration may be relevant for understanding the other as well.

Table 3.1

Risk factors common to most forms of violence
Individual factors
Positive beliefs about aggression
Insecure or anxious attachment
Anger/hostility
Emotional reactivity
Impulsivity/lack of self-control
Antisocial/aggressive behavior
Jealousy
Personality disorder
Psychopathology
Alcohol or drug abuse
Demographic factors
Young age
Low Education
Low Income
*Historical factors
Experiencing child maltreatment
Witnessing violence in family of origin
Relationship factors
Low Relationship satisfaction
High Level of conflict
Social and community factors
Life stress
Unemployment
Proximity to violent individuals
Exposure to high-risk settings
Chronic community disorder
Lack of social integration

*A childhood history of violence is one of the strongest and best known risk factors for virtually every form of violence, but of course this also fits as part of the co-occurrence framework, as a pattern of re-victimization or the origin of a perpetrator-victim dynamic

Conceptual models that can account for interconnections between different forms of violence need to integrate the wide range of constructs that have been identified as risk or vulnerability factors for both perpetration and victimization (see Table 3.1). Socio ecological perspectives (Bronfenbrenner 1977) offer one framework for organizing diverse risk factors. This type of model conceptualizes violence as occurring within a context of multiple, nested sources of influence (e.g., individual, dyadic, family, neighborhood, community, and culture), and has been applied to several forms of violence. Social ecological models, however, tend not to focus on *how* factors interact to produce violent behavior, and thus may be less helpful in identifying the causal pathways that lead to violence.

An approach that is more amenable to explicating the processes that lead to violence begins by organizing risk factors into characteristics of the person and characteristics of the situation (Bushman and Huesmann 2010; DeWall et al. 2011; Finkel 2008; Riggs and O'Leary 1996). In these models, the probability of aggressive behavior occurring at a particular moment is viewed as the product of qualities of individuals that make them more or less likely to engage in violent behavior and qualities of the situation that are more or less likely to elicit aggressive behavior. Conceptualizing potential etiological processes in terms of *who* is likely to be violent and *when* violence is more likely to occur offers a way to understand connections across different forms of interpersonal violence as well as more unique influences. Individuals vary on both intrapersonal characteristics and their exposure to situations that pull for violence, and, in general, the more pervasive and stable these person and situation factors are, the more co-occurrence would be expected. As we describe below, however, particular aspects of these processes have implications for what types of perpetration or victimization would be expected to occur, and the specific constellation of person and situation factors together would define a profile of risk for a given individual. Although both person and situation factors contribute to most violent incidents, their relative impact varies: some situations pull for aggressive behavior and consequently minimize the role of person factors (e.g., retaliating when attacked), whereas aggression in more benign or ambiguous situations is shaped to a greater extent by personal characteristics.

Theories of diverse forms of violence perpetration, particularly in psychology, consistently identify particular classes of individual characteristics as causal factors: cognitions, emotions, self-regulatory capacities, personality characteristics, and biological processes. Although specific models emphasize somewhat different factors, there is sufficient empirical evidence supporting the inclusion of each in a comprehensive framework. Situational influences have received less attention in psychological models of perpetration, but play a salient role in sociological theories. They can include a large range of factors, from broad forces such as poverty, to characteristics of communities and neighborhoods, to the behavior of others in an interaction.

Person and situation factors also can be applied to models of victimization, though situational factors usually will have a more potent effect. For example, Routine Activities Theory (Wittebrood and Nieuwbeerta 2000) conceptualizes violent victimization as shaped largely by demographic (e.g., SES, gender), family, and peer factors that result in the victim spending more time in dangerous contexts where victimization is more likely to occur. However, personal characteristics that can influence the likelihood of becoming victimized must be considered as well. Discussing individual factors related to victimization is sometimes viewed as victim blaming, but identifying personal characteristics or behaviors that increase the risk of victimization is not the same as holding an individual responsible for being victimized. There is ample evidence across forms of violence that victimization is not randomly distributed; for example, some children are more likely to be bullied than others (Card 2011) and some women are at greater risk for sexual victimization than others (Messman-Moore and Long 2003). Understanding why some individuals are viewed as "easy targets" or are more vulnerable to physical or sexual threats has critical implications for preventing victimization. Criminologists speak of "hardening the target", which involves developing strategies for making potential victims less vulnerable to perpetrators (Podolefsky and Dubow 1981), and the study of victim characteristics can be viewed similarly. Indeed, this logic is a cornerstone of prevention programs designed to reduce physical and sexual aggression in adolescence and adulthood (e.g., Foshee et al. 2009).

In the next section, we outline a heuristic framework that integrates common factors identified in prior theoretical work on violence and draws from two conceptual models that describe processes by which the interaction of person and situation factors lead to aggressive behavior: the General Aggression Model (GAM; Anderson and Bushman 2002) and the I^3 model (Finkel 2007). Both models integrate multiple levels of analysis and can be flexibly applied to different forms of violence. Although they were designed to explain the perpetration of violence, we discuss how they offer insights on victimization as well.

As its name indicates, the General Aggression Model describes processes proposed to be instrumental in the perpetration of all forms of violence. It identifies distal factors (e.g., biological processes, environmental stressors) that shape personality, which in turn interacts with situational characteristics to guide cognitions, affect, and behavior in a social interaction. Although emotions and physiological arousal are proposed to influence individuals' perceptions and responses, GAM places particular emphasis on cognitive processes such as appraisal and decision making as proximal causes of behavior. Because it is intended to be broadly applicable to different kinds of interpersonal perpetration, it does not specify the particular cognitions, emotions, physiological processes, or experiences believed to be critical for specific types.

The I^3 model was designed to understand intimate partner violence perpetration, but the processes it describes can be applied to other kinds of aggression and abuse as well. The "I"s in the I^3 model stand for "Instigating Triggers", "(Violence-)Impelling Forces", and "(Violence-)Inhibiting Forces" (Finkel 2008). Like the GAM, the I^3 model identifies individual, situational, and relational factors that make aggressive behavior more likely to occur, but in contrast to most perpetration models, it also pays equal attention to the factors that prevent violent impulses from being expressed. Finkel (2008) argues that aggressive impulses are common in close relationships because they involve high levels of emotional investment and interdependence; conflict, frustration, and perceptions of criticism or rejection arouse strong emotions in these "high-stakes" relationships, and occasionally lead to a desire to strike out against the partner. The fact that these impulses are effectively contained in most situations highlights the importance of understanding the individual, situational, and relational factors that inhibit violent behavior.

In the next section, we discuss person and situational factors that have been identified in theories of diverse forms of interpersonal violence (see Fig. 3.1) and examine how they may explain the co-occurrence of violence across contexts as well as the occurrence of isolated experiences of perpetration or victimization. We pay particular attention to the roles that these factors play in instigating, impelling, or inhibiting aggression.

person & situational factors

Individual Factors

Evidence that individual differences in aggression remain fairly stable over the lifespan (see Development chapter) and that individuals who engage in one type of violence often engage in others (see Epidemiology chapter) underscore the role of individual characteristics in explaining violent behavior. The most prominent models of the perpetration of interpersonal violence highlight the role of cognitive factors in driving aggressive behavior, but emotions, self-regulatory processes, personality traits, and biological factors also are important to include in a comprehensive understanding of the perpetration of violence.

Cognitive Processes

Cognitive theorists have identified several cognitive processes that are associated with aggression and violence. Nearly all of the studies of cognitive factors have focused on single forms of violence, but the mechanisms described in these models are likely to apply broadly across relationship contexts, and thus are essential for understanding interconnections among different types of violence. Some of these models, such as social learning theory, emphasize how past experiences with violence directly shape cognitions in ways that make further involvement in violence more likely. Others, such as the internal working models of attachment theory, place more emphasis on factors such as the quality and stability of relationships with caregivers and how these can create heightened risks for both perpetration and victimization. We highlight some of the most important cognitive models below.

Social Learning Theory has been the dominant psychological theory applied to the perpetration of a variety of forms of interpersonal violence, and the mechanisms that it proposes primarily are cognitive in nature. Social Learning Theory (Bandura 1986) holds that children learn to be aggressive by observing powerful and valued individuals (such as parents and peers) engage in aggression (i.e., modeling), particularly if the aggressive behavior results in a positive outcome for the aggressor (i.e., vicarious reinforcement). Exposure to violence (as a victim or witness) is proposed to lead to the development of beliefs that violence is normative, justifiable, and effective, and these beliefs in turn increase the likelihood of engaging in aggression toward others, both in childhood and later in life. Documented associations between aggressive beliefs and violent perpetration in several relationship contexts support this proposition (e.g., Foshee et al. 1999; Kinsfogel and Grych 2004). Aggressive beliefs also can be reinforced directly, as Capaldi et al. (2001) illustrated in a study of conversations between antisocial youths and a same-sex friend. They found that sexist and derogatory comments about females were consistently affirmed by peers in the context of these affiliative and supportive interactions.

Social Learning Theory offers a mechanism for explaining links between being a victim or witness of violence in childhood and perpetrating aggression toward peers, romantic partners, and offspring. However, we know little about how closely related beliefs about aggression in different contexts are; people may have general attitudes about the justifiability or appropriateness of aggressive behavior and context-specific beliefs as well. For example, someone may generally disapprove of the use of violence in most relationships but still endorse spanking as a means of discipline for children. Others may have more generally pro-violent attitudes or accept specific justifications, such as saving face, that will be relevant in multiple settings and relationships. Further, there has been little empirical study of the actual consequences of aggressive behavior and how they shape beliefs and later behavior. Research on how the outcome of aggression in one domain (e.g., family) predicts attitudes and behavior in that domain and in others (e.g., peer and romantic relationships) will provide tests for social learning processes.

The principles of social learning theory have been expanded and elaborated by other theorists to focus on what is learned from experiences with abuse and violence and how it affects later behavior. For example, Huesmann (1998) emphasized the role of schemas and scripts in guiding behavior. More complex than beliefs, schemas are organized "clusters" of information, attitudes, and expectations pertaining to particular situations; scripts are similar but add a temporal element that reflects the general sequence of events likely to occur in a particular situation, potential responses, and the possible consequences of those responses. These cognitive representations are proposed to affect how individuals perceive and respond to others in interpersonal interactions.

Consistent with Social Learning Theory, schemas and scripts are held to be the product of experience. Children exposed to aggression in the family, between peers, or in the community are predicted to develop expectations about interpersonal relationships and about how others are likely to treat them, as they strive to understand their experiences (DeBoard-Lucas and Grych 2011). As a result, they tend to anticipate hostility or threat from others and enter social interactions prepared to defend themselves or establish dominance. The behaviors that flow from these cognitive processes tend to elicit the hostility that they expect from others, thus confirming their schemas and creating situations in which aggression is more likely to occur.

The construct of *internal working models*, drawn from attachment theory, bears striking similarity to schemas (see Bretherton and Munholland 1999). Like schemas, working models are mental representations built from experience, but have broader relevance for understanding how individuals view the self and others in close relationships. Individuals with secure attachment styles have positive images of themselves as worthy of love and others as trustworthy and responsive, whereas insecure attachment involves views of the self as inadequate or unlovable and others as unreliable, indifferent, or rejecting (Bartholomew and Horowitz 1991). Bowlby (1969, 1973) proposed that working models are initially based on children's early interactions with their caregivers but continue to shape and be shaped by other experiences in intimate relationships throughout life. As we discuss in Chap. 4, disruptions in attachment are implicated in the early emergence of aggressive behavior and related to diverse forms of perpetration and victimization, including child abuse, exposure to family violence, teen dating violence, and adult intimate partner violence (Grych and Kinsfogel 2010). Mental representations of close relationships (schemas, working models) thus provide a thread for connecting experiences with violence across contexts and across the lifespan, and between perpetration and victimization.

Information processing models. Whereas work on schemas focuses primarily on the content of cognition—*what* people believe or expect—Dodge and colleagues' influential social information processing model (e.g., Crick and Dodge 1994) describes cognitive processes proposed to occur during aggressive interactions; i.e., *how* people think, perceive, and process information. This model was developed to understand aggressive peer interactions in childhood, but can be applied to interpersonal violence more generally (DeWall et al. 2011). It proposes that aggressive children tend to encode ambiguous social cues as threatening, attribute hostile intent to others, and more readily access and positively evaluate aggressive behavioral responses. The nature of children's information processing in a given situation is believed to be influenced by mental representations of their prior experiences. Thus, information processing offers another theoretical mechanism for explaining how early exposure to abuse and violence leads to later aggressive behavior. For example, children who were physically abused may develop the belief that other people often engage in hurtful behavior, and subsequently are more likely to perceive ambiguous behavior as threatening and view others as intending to cause them harm. Information processing would explain re-victimization and re-perpetration in similar ways. As these examples suggest, other experiences that teach children that ambiguous situations are threatening, such as growing up in a family or community that promotes distrust of outsiders, could also lead to cognitive processes that increase the risk of perpetration.

Although these cognitive processes can be consciously accessed, they often operate outside of conscious awareness. Especially, in the midst of an emotionally arousing social interaction, individuals tend not to systematically evaluate others' motives and then draw a reasoned conclusion. Rather, the process of accessing and acting on schematic information is automatic and can drive behavior without conscious attention. The distinction between automatic and controlled processing has been explored extensively in cognitive and social psychology (Chen and Chaiken 1999; Wegner and Bargh 1998). *Controlled* processing is conscious, intentional, and requires attention and cognitive resources. In contrast, *automatic* processing proceeds outside of conscious awareness, requires little effort or cognitive resources, and operates much more rapidly.

Two decades of research in cognitive and social psychology have shown that automatic processes have pervasive effects on a range of phenomena, including perception, affect, memory, judgment, problem solving, and behavior (for a review see Bargh 1997). Nonconscious processes are particularly relevant for understanding reactive aggression because of their role in guiding behavior "in the heat of the moment." Individuals vary in the ease with which particular beliefs or ideas come to mind, or their accessibility, in addition to the content of their cognitions. When aggressive thoughts are highly accessible, individuals are more likely to interpret ambiguous situational cues as aggressive or provocative, and are primed to engage in aggressive behavior (Anderson and Bushman 2002; Berkowitz 2008; Todorov and Bargh 2002). Because automatic processing is faster than controlled processing, it may lead to aggressive behavior before individuals can consciously consider their alternatives. Thus, automatic cognitions can be powerful impelling forces for perpetration. Recently, more attention has been paid to the role of automatic or nonconscious cognitive processes in driving aggressive behavior (Gilbert and Daffern 2011; Jouriles et al. 2011; Todorov and Bargh 2002). For example, Jouriles et al. (2011) reported that both the accessibility of aggressive thoughts and explicit beliefs about the consequences of dating aggression were concurrently associated with teen dating violence, but only accessibility predicted increases in aggressive behavior over the course of 3 months.

A potentially important cognitive construct that has received relatively little attention in theories of perpetration is the *goals* that individuals have in the situation (Rose and Asher 1999; Simon et al. 2008). Even reactive aggression is goal driven, though the goal(s) may not be conscious at the time the behavior occurs. People typically have multiple goals in interpersonal situations that vary in immediacy and salience and these goals could serve as either impelling or inhibiting forces. For example, during a conflict in an intimate relationship, individuals may want to win the argument, preserve the relationship, defend their self-esteem, or exert dominance. These goals are likely to lead to very different kinds of behavior, whereas a desire to dominate might impel aggression, the goal of preserving the relationship is likely to inhibit it. The salience of each goal can be shaped by person and situation factors. For example, stable intrapersonal characteristics, such as narcissism, may make defending self-worth an important goal in multiple situations, or situational factors may highlight one goal over the others. In combination with other personal characteristics such as impulsivity or poor emotion regulation, pursuing this goal may "short-circuit" more planful, controlled processing and lead the individual to strike out at their partner.

Cognition and victimization. Most of the work on cognitive processes has focused on perpetration, but there is evidence for their relevance for victimization as well. The belief that violence is a normative or acceptable part of close relationships may lead individuals to tolerate aggression from an intimate partner. Self-representations also may be related to victimization. For example, children who are bullied tend to report lower self-efficacy for assertive behavior and to believe that seeking help from teachers will make their situation worse rather than better (Camodeca and Goossens 2005; Egan and Perry 1998). Consequently, they may be perceived by others as an "easy target", because they are unlikely to defend themselves or do something that will lead to negative consequences for the aggressor. In the domain of sexual violence, it has been proposed that cognitive appraisals and emotions influence women's behavioral responses to attempted sexual assault (Nurius and Norris 1996). Nurius and colleagues have shown that several types of cognitions, including the desire to preserve the relationship and concerns about being judged negatively by the male, predicted how assertively women responded to attempted sexual assaults (Macy et al. 2006; Nurius et al. 2004).

Social cognitive models are valuable for understanding both the co-occurrence of violence in different contexts and specific forms of aggression. From this perspective, the cognitive processes described above combine to shape the meaning of a particular event to individuals and the repertoire of responses they believe will be effective or appropriate in the situation. If abuse and harm are salient aspects of individuals' schemas for interpersonal relationships, they are likely to be sensitive to threat cues and perceive threat across multiple situations whether a particular type of violence is likely to occur depends on the content of individuals' schemas and scripts, the existence of particular types of beliefs and goals, and salient features of the situation. For example, individuals who believe that hitting is a normative and effective way to exact compliance from a disobedient child would be at increased risk for perpetrating child abuse. If their schemas for adult intimate relationships similarly involve the belief that it is justifiable to physically dominate their partner when they are in conflict, co-occurrence of child maltreatment and partner abuse might be expected. In contrast, if their schemas for intimate relationships involve a more egalitarian balance of power and different strategies for resolving difficulties with a partner as opposed to a child, they might aggress against a child but be unlikely to aggress against their partner. Although other factors also impel or inhibit aggressive behavior, these models suggest that the content of cognition plays a role in determining in which situations interpersonal violence is likely to be perpetrated.

Emotional Processes

The amount of attention paid to cognitive processes in theory and research on aggression reflects the dominant influence of Social Learning Theory, but underplays the extent to which emotions also shape the meaning of situations and drive behavior. Interpersonal relationships elicit strong emotions, because they are a primary context for meeting essential human needs for affiliation, self-esteem, and nurturance. Threats to these needs can generate powerful emotional responses and give rise to violent behavior. In fact, one of the earliest psychological theories of aggression conceptualized it as a response to emotion. The Frustration-Aggression hypothesis (Dollard et al. 1939) held that frustration arises when important goals are blocked, and this unpleasant affective state then motivates aggressive behavior in an attempt to remove the obstacle. Recognition that frustration can lead to behaviors other than aggression and that aggression can occur in the absence of frustration led this theory to fall out of favor (Bushman and Huesmann 2010), but the premise that aggression often is a motivated response to anger and frustration has been supported by more recent work.

Contemporary developmental and clinical theories have conceptualized anger as a natural (i.e., unlearned) response to the perception that someone or something is blocking an important goal, threatening one's well-being, or violating a valued moral principle (Stein and Levine 1987; Stein and Liwag 1997). From this perspective, aggression represents an effort to remove the obstacle, and thus reinstate the goal (i.e., protect the self from violation, right the "wrong"). For example, the perception that one's partner is having an affair threatens an important goal (being in the relationship) and so is likely to produce anger. The view of aggression as goal-driven behavior spurred by anger is supported by research showing that the tendency to experience and express higher levels of anger consistently predicts perpetration in adult (Norlander and Eckhardt 2005; O'Leary et al. 2007) and adolescent intimate relationships (Kinsfogel and Grych 2004; Wolfe et al. 1998).Threats to the self or important goals can elicit other emotions as well (e.g., fear) and may give rise to responses other than aggression; thus, the relations between emotions and the perpetration of violence can be complex.

How anger and other emotions are expressed also is a function of individuals' capacity to regulate affect. Individuals with emotion regulation problems are more likely to become upset and act on aggressive impulses in a variety of interpersonal situations (Feiring et al. 2002; Fosco et al. 2007; Stuewig and McCloskey 2005). Emotion regulation capacities undoubtedly have a biological basis, but experience can affect them as well. For example, child maltreatment and exposure to interparental aggression are associated with poor emotion regulation (Davies and Cummings 1998; Fosco and Grych 2008; Gratz et al. 2009; Maughan and Cicchetti 2002).

Emotion constructs rarely have been included in models of victimization. The sexual victimization model developed by Nurius and Norris (1996) described above is one exception. Consistent with the idea that aggression can be an adaptive response to threats to the self, they found that women experiencing anger during attempted sexual assaults were more likely to engage in assertive behavior (Nurius et al. 2004). High levels of fear, in contrast, could be immobilizing and interfere with effective behavioral responses.

Both the tendency to experience anger and difficulties with regulating emotion are critical for explaining why violence occurs in multiple relationship contexts. The I^3 framework identifies feelings of anger as a key trigger for perpetration and the general capacity for modulating emotion as an inhibiting force that decreases aggression across contexts. Thus, tendencies to experience and have difficulty regulating anger in a variety of interpersonal contexts can help to explain the interconnections among different forms of violence.

Emotions arise from the subjective meaning of a situation, which is shaped by prior experiences and intrapersonal characteristics as well as the nature of the interaction. Consequently, some individuals are more likely to experience anger–and engage in aggression–across contexts. For example, individuals who are highly sensitive to criticism often may feel "attacked" by others and become angry and aggressive whenever they feel slighted. They might be expected to exhibit aggression in multiple relationships. In contrast, individuals who have anxious attachment styles are prone to perceiving rejection in intimate relationships and may strike out when they perceive that a relationship is threatened (Grych and Kinsfogel 2010); however, they may exhibit aggression only in those relationships. There also may be individual differences in the propensity to experience particular emotions. Jenkins and Oatley (1997) proposed that exposure to hostility and violence in the family may organize children's emotions around anger, making it the default response to upsetting stimuli even in situations when anger is not typically elicited (Jenkins 2000; Jenkins and Oatley 1997).

Self-Regulation

Emotion regulation reflects one facet of self-regulation, which typically is conceptualized more broadly as management of behavior in the service of a goal. Self-regulation involves eliciting and maintaining an adaptive level of arousal, modulating affect, and inhibiting impulses that would interfere with goal-directed behavior. These processes are hypothesized to have their basis in neuropsychological processes involved in executive functioning. Self-regulation has had a prominent role in theories of aggression. In the criminology literature, self-control theory (Gottfredson and Hirschi 1990) holds that the capacity to inhibit aggressive impulses is central to explaining violent crime, and has been supported by an extensive series of studies (for a meta-analytic review see Pratt and Cullen 2000). The inverse of self-control, impulsivity, also has been consistently associated with aggressive and violent behavior (e.g., Frick and Hare 2001), and is particularly relevant for understanding reactive aggression. The behavior of impulsive or poorly self-regulated individuals is more influenced by automatic cognitive processes; these individuals tend to act without reflection, and thus impulses that might be inhibited by controlled reasoning are enacted before their potential consequences can be evaluated.

Self-regulation is the centerpiece of the I^3 model, which views self-control as a product of person and situational factors. In an elegant series of studies, Finkel and colleagues showed that adults could better inhibit aggressive impulses during conflict when they exhibited higher levels of dispositional self-control, were not under time pressure to respond, and received training designed to bolster self-regulation (Finkel et al. 2009). Thus, although self-regulatory capacity has trait-like characteristics that evidence stability from childhood through adolescence (Hay and Forrest 2006), individuals' ability to manage aggressive impulses in a given situation can be influenced by a range of factors. Whereas consistently poor self-regulation can help explain co-occurrence of perpetration across relationships, even characteristically strong self-regulatory skills can be undermined under certain conditions.

Personality

The self-regulatory, cognitive, and emotional processes discussed above can be conceptualized as personality characteristics, because they represent enduring patterns of thinking, feeling, and behaving. More traditional, trait-oriented approaches to personality also have identified several characteristics that are consistently linked to violence. Because personality characteristics generally are viewed as stable and pervasive, they are likely to play a significant role in causing the co-occurrence of violence across contexts and relationships.

The personality traits that are most relevant for understanding violence are those that have an impelling or inhibiting effect on aggressive behavior, and psychopathy is the trait most often associated with antisocial and aggressive behavior. Psychopathy has several components that may function to impel violent perpetration in different ways: impulsivity, callous/unemotional traits, and narcissism. Callous/unemotional traits reflect lack of empathy, lack of guilt, and use of others for one's own ends (Frick and White 2008). This component of psychopathy is fairly stable across the lifespan (e.g., Frick et al. 2003) and appears to distinguish more and less violent forms of conduct disorder in youths and to differentiate adults higher in psychopathy from other antisocial adults. Antisocial youth who are high in callous/unemotional traits exhibit cognitive and emotional qualities that suggest that they are less sensitive to and less distressed by the consequences of their behavior, both for themselves and others (Frick and White 2008). They are less sensitive to fear and distress, less fearful of punishment, and express lower levels of anxiety and higher levels of fearlessness. They also evaluate aggressive behavior more positively than children who are lower in these traits. Empathy for others is an important violence-inhibiting force, and tends to be stronger in close relationships. Having low levels of empathy removes a powerful brake on aggressive impulses, and would be expected to result in greater likelihood of violent behavior across contexts and relationships.

Narcissism consistently predicts aggressive behavior in naturalistic and laboratory studies, in children and adolescents, and toward peers and dating partners (Kerig and Stellwagen 2010; Ryan et al. 2008; Thomaes et al. 2008). Narcissism can be conceptualized as self-aggrandizement that functions as a defense against low self-worth; individuals high in narcissism are exceptionally sensitive to criticism and often perceive benign behaviors as a threat to their self-esteem, and thus frequently feel attacked by others. They lash out verbally or physically in an attempt to strike back at those they perceive as hurting them, or to regain a sense of dominance. This hypersensitivity to threats to their self-esteem likely cuts across relationships and so could lead to different forms of aggression, but may be especially keen in intimate relationships where the emotional "stakes" are higher.

Biological Factors

In the last 10 years, interest has surged in genetic and biological factors related to violence. There is evidence that aggression has a strong genetic component (Miles and Carey 1997; Moffitt 2005), but the pathways through which genes lead to aggressive behavior are less clear (Raine 2008). Several candidates for physiological mediators have been identified (e.g., prefrontal cortex, amygdala, serotonin, and HPA axis) that suggest at least two primary influences on behavior. First, underarousal in key neurological structures and processes may reduce individuals' sensitivity to punishment or other consequences of their behavior, which in turn reduces the influence of the inhibiting forces that typically constrain aggressive impulses (e.g., Raine et al. 1995). Underarousal thus may provide a biological basis for callous/unemotional traits and impulsivity. Second, dysregulation in the biological stress response may undermine adaptive responses to events and interactions that elicit physiological arousal (e.g., Susman 2006). The behavioral manifestation of this process may be in the form of poor emotion and self-regulation in threatening or stressful situations, both of which could increase the likelihood of either perpetration or victimization.

Both underarousal and dysregulated responses to stress would be expected to have pervasive effects on aggressive behavior, and thus may contribute to understanding the co-occurrence of different forms of violence. Biological processes also represent one of the few domains in which similar processes have been identified to account for victimization and perpetration of aggression. Research on child maltreatment and exposure to violence suggests that they may have common effects on the functioning of the human stress response (Cicchetti and Rogosch 2001; Saltzman et al. 2005), which involves the sympathetic and parasympathetic nervous systems, neurotransmitters, and the hypothalamic–pituitary–adrenal (HPA) axis (De Bellis 2001; Watts-English et al. 2006). When exposed to chronic or repeated stress, this system may fail to return to baseline and become dysregulated when the individuals are faced with later stressors (Susman 2006). This in turn may undermine their capacity to control aggressive impulses, and also may place them at greater risk for victimization. Noll and Grych (2011) developed a model of sexual revictimization that centers on this process. They proposed that sexual abuse in childhood leads to hyperarousal of the HPA axis, which in turn dysregulates the cognitive, physiological, and emotional processes needed to engage in effective responses to sexual threats. Over time, the stress response becomes attenuated, impairing females' ability to mobilize assertive resistance behavior. The effects of early victimization may well be broader than this, however, and may extend to other types of exposure to violence in childhood and to perpetration of violence as well as victimization.

Situational Factors

Because different types of violence by definition involve different situations, situational factors would appear to be more important for understanding specificity than generality in experiences with violence perpetration or victimization. However, there are at least two reasons why attention to situational factors can contribute to understanding the co-occurrence of violence. First, as suggested by routine activities theory (Wittebrood and Nieuwbeerta 2000), there can be consistencies in the kinds of situations that people encounter. Certain types of activities, such as going out to bars at night, will likely bring individuals into contact with more perpetrators or potential perpetrators and are associated with higher victimization risk (Sampson and Lauritsen 1993). A variety of social, economic, and individual factors can result in repeated exposure to settings in which violence is more likely to occur (Sampson and Lauritsen 1993). For example, individuals low in socioeconomic status tend to live in more dangerous neighborhoods where crime is more likely to occur, and face chronic stressors that increase the risk of intimate partner violence and child maltreatment. There also may be similarities in the people that individuals interact with. Aggressive people have a tendency to associate with peers who also are more aggressive than average (Pepler et al. 2008), which increases the chance that hostile and violent situations will arise.

A variety of environmental and community-level factors have been identified as risk factors for violence perpetration, victimization, or both. As with person factors, they may serve as triggers, impelling forces, or inhibitors of aggression. Aversive events that produce irritability, frustration, rejection, and other unpleasant mood states create the potential for aggressive behavior (Berkowitz 1989; Bushman and Huesmann 2010). These can include environmental conditions such as temperature, crowding, and buildings that have fallen into disrepair (DeWall et al. 2011; Sampson and Lauritsen 1993). For example, the "broken windows" theory (Kelling and Coles 1996) suggests that neglected neighborhood environments (in terms of upkeep and cleanliness) promote criminal behavior. The availability of weapons, alcohol, and drugs can both increase the level of threat and danger present in the environment and affect how individuals respond to perceived threats. Alcohol and drug use can increase perpetration, particularly in those more prone to aggression, by elevating physiological arousal, reducing behavioral inhibition, and impairing judgment. Substance use is also a risk for victimization as it can reduce a person's ability to identify risky situations and protect oneself from potential attacks. Chronic exposure to violent or intensely competitive media, including video games, television, and movies, may also be associated with aggression (Adachi and Willoughby 2011; Bushman and Huesmann 2010). A variety of structural and cultural conditions are associated with increased risks of violence, including poverty, unemployment, residential mobility, and subcultural values (Goodman et al. 2009; Sampson and Lauritsen 1993; Wolfgang and Ferracuti 1967).

The nature of individuals' social relationships also can influence the occurrence of violence. Scholars have pointed to the degree to which individuals are "socially integrated" as a major inhibiting force for numerous types of aggression, ranging from intimate partner violence (Ramirez 2007) to street crime (Gottfredson and Hirschi 1990). Lack of social integration is also thought to be one of the mechanisms by which factors such as chronic unemployment increase risk of perpetration. Beyond the individual level, collective efficacy, which embodies the shared expectations for social control, social cohesion, and trust in a community, is also associated with rates of violence (Sampson et al. 1997). However, the most direct interpersonal influence on violence comes from the behavior of other people present in the situation.

The Behavior of Others

Each person in an interaction can serve as an instigating trigger for the other, and can either impel or inhibit violence. Interpersonal interactions perceived to be hostile, provocative, or rejecting have the potential to evoke negative affect and aggressive impulses (Bushman and Huesmann 2010). Such interactions also reinforce existing aggressogenic beliefs and schemas. Research on parent–child and marital interactions shows that violence often is the culmination of an escalating series of behaviors that become increasingly hostile or conflictual. The importance of dyadic interactions in relationships also is underscored by data showing that the stability of an individual's violence toward their partner is fairly high when they remain in the same relationship and much smaller with a different partner (Capaldi et al. 2003; Williams et al. 2008). Similarly, Card (2011) has noted that the majority of aggression in peer relationships occurs within specific bully-victim dyads. The behavior of others in the social environment also can affect whether violence occurs. For example, other children can influence whether bullying occurs by encouraging or discouraging fighting between two potential combatants. This observation has led to the development of prevention programs that try to reduce violence by increasing intervention by bystanders (Banyard 2011).

Several models have been developed recently that place more emphasis on the interaction between individuals in explaining violence. For example, Capaldi et al. (2005) argue that the prediction of intimate partner violence requires attention to the individual characteristics of each person in the relationship, including their personality, psychopathology, and developmental stage, as well as situational factors. O'Leary and Slep (2003) developed a similar model to explain the occurrence of aggression in adolescent dating relationships. In the domain of bullying, Card (2011) integrated social-cognitive theory with interdependence theory in order to describe how the cognitions and behavior of both bully and victim contribute to the aggression that occurs in the relationship. All of these models speak to the power of situational factors in shaping violence. The nature of the relationship itself also may play a role.

The Relationship Context

The relationship context refers to the type of relationship in which violence occurs (e.g. parent–child, peer, intimate partner) and its status (how close or committed the relationship is). Relationships differ substantially in the needs that they fulfill, the level of investment or commitment they involve, and what is "at stake" in them. These needs and their associated goals play important roles in shaping the meaning of particular situations. For example, close relationships evoke attachment needs, along with their associated beliefs and expectations, and become more important to individuals than more casual friendships. Consequently, a critical comment from an acquaintance may be shrugged off, but the same comment by an intimate partner may cut deeply and elicit pain and anger. Understanding why interpersonal violence occurs thus involves attending to how particular relationship contexts influence individuals' perceptions of self and other, and both shape and are shaped by individuals' goals and needs.

In general, the risk of violence increases as relationships become more serious; indicators of relationship seriousness such as duration, emotional commitment, and physical intimacy all predict greater violence in dating relationships (Halpern et al. 2001; O'Keefe and Treister 1998). Violence also is more common in relationships that involve frequent conflict and power struggles (Bentley et al. 2007; O'Keefe

1997). Early in a new relationship, there tends to be less conflict as individuals identify common interests and focus on the positive aspects of the relationship; the desire to present a good impression also may override impulses toward anger that do arise. When relationship intimacy and investment increase, so do the emotional "stakes" and potential threats to the relationships take on more importance. Individuals also face decisions that may lead to conflict or power struggles (e.g., to see others or not, to become more committed or not), resentment, and jealousy. From an attachment perspective, as dating relationships become more serious, they take on attachment functions (e.g., reliance on partner for acceptance, distress over separation; Furman and Collins 2009). Consequently, the potential loss of the relationship may become more threatening, which may lead to control or abusive behavior intended to keep the partner close. The break-up of a relationship also is a particularly high-risk time for violence (Tjaden and Thoennes 2000).

Card's (2011) relational model of bullying also highlights the importance of considering the nature of the relationship between perpetrators and victims. Although nearly all of the work on bullying has focused on identifying individual differences that characterize bullies (or subtypes of bullies) and victims, the finding that the majority of bullying in a peer group occurs between a small number of specific dyads brings attention to the role of relationship factors. This model identifies relationship-specific cognitions that may explain why a particular bully picks on a particular victim, and considers how victims' responses to early bullying behaviors influence whether the bully-victim relationship continues or not. A similar dynamic might occur in romantic relationships.

Whether increasing closeness leads to conflict or aggression in a particular relationship in turn may be best explained by considering the characteristics that each person brings to the relationship and their interaction. Capaldi et al. (2005) have proposed a dyadic model of intimate partner violence that highlights the roles of particular qualities of couples' interaction (e.g., conflict resolution), the proximal context in which interactions occur (e.g., use of drugs or alcohol), and the developmental history of each partner (including personality and psychopathology). The few studies examining aggression in adolescent relationships provide empirical support for including characteristics of the relationship or partner as predictors. For example, Cano et al. (1998) showed that the level of aggression reported by adolescents was predicted both by their prior aggressive/antisocial behavior and the behavior of their partner, and O'Leary and Slep (2003) found that youths' level of aggressive behavior at Time 1 no longer predicted aggression at Time 2 once their partner's behavior was included as a predictor.

Conclusion

Our discussion of theoretical models of violence indicates that many of the proposed causes of aggression are common to different forms of abuse and violence, and suggests that these processes represent one important source of co-occurrence.

In particular, personality characteristics, emotion and self-regulation, and genetic/biological factors are likely to have pervasive effects on behavior across contexts. Cognitive constructs and processes, in contrast, vary in their generality and consequently could lead to both poly- and mono-perpetration and victimization. Although situational factors are more likely to account for specificity in perpetration and victimization, some are consistent across multiple relationship contexts (e.g., poverty, neighborhood characteristics) and so can contribute to co-occurrence as well. Given that experiences with violence, abuse, and trauma can produce many of the processes identified as causes of violence, they represent another source for the covariation among different forms. In the next chapter, we examine developmental processes that shape the cognitive, affective, and biological processes described above, and pay particular attention to the impact of violence on these processes.

References

Adachi, P., & Willoughby, T. (2011). The effect of video game competition and violence on aggressive behavior: Which characteristic has the greatest influence? *Psychology of Violence, 1*(4), 259–274.

Anderson, C. A., & Bushman, B. J. (2002). Human aggression. *Annual Review of Psychology, 53*, 27–51.

Bandura, A. (1986). *Social foundations of thought and action: A social cognitive theory.* Englewood Cliffs: Prentice Hall.

Banyard, V. (2011). Who will help prevent sexual violence: Creating an ecological model of bystander intervention. *Psychology of Violence, 1*(3), 216–229.

Bargh, J. A. (1997). The automaticity of everyday life. In R. Wyer (Ed.), *The automaticity of everyday life: Advances in social cognition* (Vol. 10, pp. 1–61). Mahwah: Erlbaum.

Bartholomew, K., & Horowitz, L. (1991). Attachment styles among young adults: A test of a four category model. *Journal of Personality and Social Psychology, 61*, 226–244.

Bentley, C., Galliher, R., & Ferguson, T. (2007). Associations among aspects of interpersonal power and relationship functioning in adolescent romantic couples. *Sex Roles, 57*, 483–495.

Berkowitz, L. (1989). The frustration-aggression hypothesis: Examination and reformulation. *Psychological Bulletin, 106*, 59–73.

Berkowitz, L. (2008). On the consideration of automatic as well as controlled psychological processes in aggression. *Aggressive Behavior, 34*(2), 117–129.

Bowlby, J. (1969). *Attachment and loss: Vol. 1. Attachment.* London: Hogarth.

Bowlby, J. (1973). *Attachment and loss: Vol. 2. Separation, anxiety and anger.* New York: Basic Books.

Bretherton, I., & Munholland, K. (1999). Internal working models in attachment: A construct revisited. In J. Cassidy & P. Shaver (Eds.), *Handbook of attachment: Theory, research and clinical application* (pp. 89–111). New York: Guilford.

Bronfenbrenner, U. (1977). Toward an experimental ecology of human development. *American Psychologist, 32*, 513–531.

Bushman, B. J., & Huesmann, L. (2010). Aggression. In S. T. Fiske, D. T. Gilbert, & G. Lindzey (Eds.), *Handbook of social psychology* (5th ed., pp. 833–863). New York: Wiley.

Camodeca, M., & Goossens, F. (2005). Aggression, social cognitions, anger and sadness in bullies and victims. *Journal of Child Psychology and Psychiatry, 46*(2), 186–197.

Cano, A., Avery-Leaf, S., Cascardi, M., & O'Leary, K. D. (1998). Dating violence in two high schools: Discriminating variables. *Journal of Primary Prevention, 18*, 431–446.

Capaldi, D., Dishion, T., Stoolmiller, M., & Yoerger, K. (2001). Aggression toward female partners by at-risk young men: The contribution of male adolescent friendships. *Developmental Psychology, 37*, 61–73.

Capaldi, D., Pears, K., Patterson, G., & Owen, L. (2003). Continuity of parenting practices across generations in an at-risk sample: A prospective comparison of direct and mediated associations. *Journal of Abnormal Child Psychology, 31*, 127–142.

Capaldi, D., Shortt, J., & Kim, H. (2005). A life span developmental systems perspective on aggression toward a partner. In W. Pinsof & J. Lebow (Eds.), *Family psychology: The art of the science* (pp. 141–167). New York: Oxford University Press.

Card, N. (2011). Toward a relationship perspective on aggression among schoolchildren: Integrating social cognitive and interdependence theories. *Psychology of Violence, 1*(3), 188–201.

Chen, S., & Chaiken, S. (1999). The heuristic-systematic model in its broader context. In S. Chaiken & Y. Trope (Eds.), *Dual-process theories in social psychology* (pp. 73–96). New York: Guilford.

Cicchetti, D., & Rogosch, F. (2001). The impact of child maltreatment and psychopathology upon neuroendocrine functioning. *Development and Psychopathology, 13*, 783–804.

Crick, N. R., & Dodge, K. (1994). A review and reformulation of social information-processing mechanisms in children's social adjustment. *Psychological Bulletin, 115*, 74–101.

Davies, P., & Cummings, E. M. (1998). Exploring children's emotional security as a mediator of the link between marital relations and child adjustment. *Child Development, 69*, 124–139.

De Bellis, M. (2001). Developmental traumatology: The psychobiological development of maltreated children and its implications for research, treatment, and policy. *Development and Psychopathology, 13*, 537–561.

DeBoard-Lucas, R., & Grych, J. H. (2011). Children's perceptions of intimate partner violence: Causes, consequences, and coping. *Journal of Family Violence, 26*(5), 343–354.

DeWall, C. N., Anderson, C. A., & Bushman, B. J. (2011). The general aggression model: Theoretical extensions to violence. *Psychology of Violence, 1*(3), 245–258.

Dollard, J., Miller, N., Doob, L., Mowrer, O., & Sears, R. (1939). *Frustration and aggression.* New Haven: Yale University Press.

Egan, S. K., & Perry, D. G. (1998). Does low self-regard invite victimization? *Developmental Psychology, 34*(2), 299–309.

Feiring, C., Deblinger, E., Hoch-Espada, A., & Haworth, T. (2002). Romantic relationship aggression and attitudes in high school students: The role of gender, grade, and attachment and emotional styles. *Journal of Youth and Adolescence, 31*(5), 373–385.

Finkel, E. (2007). Impelling and inhibiting forces in the perpetration of intimate partner violence. *Review of General Psychology, 11*, 193–207.

Finkel, E. (2008). Intimate partner violence perpetration: Insights from the science of self-regulation. In J. Forgas & J. Fitness (Eds.), *Social relationships: Cognitive, affective, and motivational processes.* New York: Psychology Press.

Finkel, E., DeWall, C. N., Slotter, E. B., Oaten, M., & Foshee, V. A. (2009). Self-regulatory failure and intimate partner violence perpetration. *Journal of Personality and Social Psychology, 97*(3), 483–499. doi:Doi10.1037/A0015433.

Fosco, G., & Grych, J. H. (2008). Integrating emotional, cognitive, and family systems mediators of children's adjustment to interparental conflict. *Journal of Family Psychology, 22*, 843–854.

Fosco, G., DeBoard, R., & Grych, J. H. (2007). Making sense of family violence: Implications of children's appraisals of interparental aggression for their short- and long-term functioning. *European Psychologist, 12*, 6–16.

Foshee, V., Bauman, K., & Linder, F. (1999). Family violence and the perpetration of adolescent dating violence: Examining social learning and social control processes. *Journal of Marriage and Family, 61*, 331–342.

Foshee, V., Reyes, H., & Wyckoff, S. C. (2009). Approaches to preventing psychological, physical, and sexual partner abuse. In K. D. O'Leary & E. Woodin (Eds.), *Understanding psychological and physical aggression in couples: Existing evidence and clinical implications.* Washington: American Psychological Association.

Frick, P., & Hare, R. (2001). *The antisocial process screening device (ASPD)*. Toronto: Multi Health Systems.

Frick, P., & White, S. F. (2008). The importance of callous-unemotional traits for developmental models of aggressive and antisocial behavior. *Journal of Child Psychology and Psychiatry, 49*(4), 359–375. doi:Doi10.1111/J.1469-7610.2007.01862.X.

Frick, P., Kimonis, E., Dandreaux, D., & Farrell, J. (2003). The four-year stability of psychopathic traits in non-referred youth. *Behavioral Sciences and the Law, 21*, 713–736.

Furman, W., & Collins, W. (2009). Adolescent romantic relationships and experiences. In K. H. Rubin, W. Bukowski, & B. Laursen (Eds.), *Peer interactions, relationships, and groups* (pp. 341–360). New York: Guilford.

Gilbert, F., & Daffern, M. (2011). Illuminating the relationship between personality disorder and violence: The contributions of the general aggression model. *Psychology of Violence, 1*(3), 230–244.

Goodman, L. A., Smyth, K. F., Borges, A. M., & Singer, R. (2009). When crises collide: How intimate partner violence and poverty intersect to shape women's mental health and coping? *Trauma, Violence, and Abuse, 10*(4), 306–329. doi:10.1177/1524838009339754.

Gottfredson, M. R., & Hirschi, T. (1990). *A general theory of crime*. Palo Alto, CA: Stanford University Press.

Gratz, K., Paulson, A., Jakupcak, M., & Tull, M. (2009). Exploring the relationship between childhood maltreatment and intimate partner abuse: Gender differences in the mediating role of emotion dysregulation. *Violence and Victims, 24*, 68–82.

Grych, J. H., & Kinsfogel, K. (2010). Exploring the role of attachment style in the relation between family aggression and abuse in adolescent dating relationships. *Journal of Aggression, Maltreatment, and Trauma, 19*, 624–664.

Halpern, C., Oslak, S., Young, M., Martin, S., & Kupper, L. (2001). Partner violence among adolescents in opposite-sex romantic relationships: Findings from the national longitudinal study of adolescent health. *American Journal of Public Health, 91*(10), 1679–1685.

Hay, C., & Forrest, W. (2006). The development of self-control: Examining self-control theory's stability thesis. *Criminology, 44*(4), 739–774.

Huesmann, L. (1998). The role of social information processing and cognitive schema in the acquisition and maintenance of habitual aggressive behavior. In R. Geen & E. Donnerstein (Eds.), *Human aggression: Theories, research, and implications for social policy* (pp. 73–109). New York: Academic Press.

Jenkins, J. (2000). Marital conflict and children's emotions: The development of an anger organization. *Journal of Marriage and the Family, 62*(3), 723–736.

Jenkins, J., & Oatley, K. (1997). The emotional brain. In J. Jenkins, K. Oatley, & N. Stein (Eds.), *Human emotions: A reader*. Malden: Blackwell.

Jouriles, E., Grych, J. H., McDonald, R., Rosenfield, D., & Dodson, M. C. (2011). Automatic cognitions and teen dating violence. *Psychology of Violence, 1*(4), 302–314. doi:10.1037/a0025157.

Kelling, G., & Coles, C. (1996). *Fixing broken windows: Restoring order and reducing crime in our communities*. New York: Touchstone.

Kerig, P., & Stellwagen, K. (2010). Roles of callous-unemotional traits, narcissism, and Machiavellianism in childhood aggression. *Journal of Psychopathology and Behavioral Assessment, 32*, 343–352.

Kinsfogel, K., & Grych, J. H. (2004). Interparental conflict and adolescent dating relationships: Integrating cognitive, emotional, and peer influences. *Journal of Family Psychology, 18*, 505–515.

Macy, R., Nurius, P., & Norris, J. (2006). Responding in their best interests: Contextualizing women's coping with acquaintance sexual aggression. *Violence against Women, 12*(5), 478–500. doi:Doi10.1177/1077801206288104.

Maughan, A., & Cicchetti, D. (2002). Impact of child maltreatment and interadult violence on children's emotion regulation abilities and socioemotional adjustment. *Child Development, 73*, 1525–1542.

Messman-Moore, T.L., & Long, P.J. (2003). The role of childhood sexual abuse sequelae in the sexual victimization of women: An empirical review and theoretical reformulation. *Clinical Psychology, 23*, 537–571.

Miles, D., & Carey, G. (1997). Genetic and environmental architecture of human aggression. *Journal of Personality and Social Psychology, 72*, 207–217.

Moffitt, T. E. (2005). The new look of behavioral genetics in developmental psychopathology. *Psychological Bulletin, 131*, 533–554.

Noll, J. G., & Grych, J. H. (2011). Read-react-respond: An integrative model for understanding sexual revictimization. *Psychology of Violence, 1*(3), 202–215.

Norlander, B., & Eckhardt, C. (2005). Anger, hostility, and male perpetrators of intimate partner violence: A meta-analytic review. *Clinical Psychology Review, 25*(2), 119–152. doi:Doi10.1016/J.Cpr.2004.10.001.

Nurius, P., & Norris, J. (1996). A cognitive-ecological of women's response to male sexual coercion in dating. *Journal of Personality and Human Sexuality, 8*, 117–139.

Nurius, P., Norris, J., Macy, R. J., & Huang, B. (2004). Women's situational coping with acquaintance sexual assault: Applying an appraisal-based model. *Violence against Women, 10*(5), 450–478. doi:Doi10.1177/1077801204264367.

O'Keefe, M., & Treister, L. (1998). Victims of dating violence among high school students: Are the predictors different for males and females? *Violence Against Women, 4*, 195–223.

O'Keefe, M. (1997). Adolescents' exposure to community and school violence: Prevalence and behavioral correlates. *Journal of Adolescent Health, 20*, 368–376.

O'Leary, K. D., & Slep, A. M. S. (2003). A dyadic longitudinal model of adolescent dating aggression. *Journal of Clinical Child and Adolescent Psychology, 32*(3), 314–327.

O'Leary, K. D., Slep, A. M. S., & O'Leary, S. G. (2007). Multivariate models of men's and women's partner aggression. *Journal of Consulting and Clinical Psychology, 75*(5), 752–764. doi:Doi10.1037/0022-006x.75.5.752.

Pepler, D., Jiang, D., Craig, W., & Connolly, J. (2008). Developmental trajectories of bullying and associated factors. *Child Development, 79*, 325–338.

Podolefsky, A., & Dubow, F. (1981). *Strategies for community crime prevention: Collective responses to crime in urban America*. Springfield: Charles C. Thomas.

Pratt, T. C., & Cullen, F. T. (2000). The empirical status of Gottfredson and Hirschi's general theory of crime: A meta-analysis. *Criminology, 38*(3), 931–964.

Raine, A. (2008). From genes to brain to antisocial behavior. *Current Directions in Psychological Science, 17*, 323–328.

Raine, A., Venables, P., & Williams, M. (1995). High autonomic arousal and electrodermal orienting at age 15 as possible protective factors against criminal behavior at age 29. *American Journal of Psychiatry, 152*, 1595–1600.

Ramirez, I. L. (2007). The relationship of acculturation and social integration to assaults on intimate partners among Mexican American and non-Mexican white students. *Journal of Family Violence, 22*, 533–542.

Riggs, D. S., & O'Leary, K. D. (1996). Aggression between heterosexual dating partners: An examination of a causal model of courtship aggression. *Journal of Interpersonal Violence, 11*, 519–540.

Rose, A., & Asher, S. (1999). Children's goals and strategies in response to conflicts within a friendship. *Developmental Psychology, 35*, 69–79.

Ryan, K., Weikel, K., & Sprechini, G. (2008). Gender differences in narcissism and courtship violence in dating couples. *Sex Roles, 58*, 802–813.

Saltzman, K., Holden, G., & Holahan, C. (2005). The psychobiology of children exposed to marital violence. *Journal of Clinical Child and Adolescent Psychology, 34*, 129–139.

Sampson, R., & Lauritsen, J. L. (1993). *Violent victimization and offending: Individual-, situational-, and community-level risk factors Understanding and preventing violence. Vol. 3, social influences* (pp. 1–114). Washington: National Academy Press.

Sampson, R., Raudenbush, S. W., & Earls, F. (1997). Neighborhoods and violent crime: A multilevel study of collective efficacy. *Science, 277*(5328), 918–924. doi:10.1126/science.277.5328.918.

Simon, V., Kobielski, S., & Martin, S. (2008). Conflict beliefs, goals, and behavior in romantic relationships during late adolescence. *Journal of Youth and Adolescence, 37*, 324–335.

Stein, N., & Levine, L. (1987). Thinking about feelings: The development and organization of emotional knowledge. In R. Snow & M. Farr (Eds.), *Aptitude, learning and instruction* (Vol. 3, pp. 165–197). Hillsdale: Erlbaum.

Stein, N., & Liwag, M. (1997). A goal-appraisal process approach to understanding and remembering emotional events. In P. van den Broek, P. Bauer & T. Bourg (Eds.), *Developmental spans in event comprehension and representation* (pp. 199–236). Hillsdale: Erlbaum.

Stuewig, J., & McCloskey, L. A. (2005). The relation of child maltreatment to shame and guilt among adolescents: Psychological routes to depression and delinquency. *Child Maltreatment, 10*(4), 324–336. doi:Doi10.1177/1077559505279308.

Susman, E. (2006). Psychobiology of persistent antisocial behavior: Stress, early vulnerabilities and the attenuation hypothesis. *Neuroscience and Biobehavioral Reviews, 30*, 376–389.

Thomaes, S., Bushman, B. J., Stegge, H., & Olthof, T. (2008). Trumping shame by blasts of noise: Narcissism, self-esteem, shame, and aggression in young adolescents. *Child Development, 79*, 1792–1801.

Tjaden, P., & Thoennes, N. (2000). *Extent, nature, and consequences of intimate partner violence: Findings from the national violence against women survey*. Washington: National Institutes of Justice.

Todorov, A., & Bargh, J. A. (2002). Automatic sources of aggression. *Aggression and Violent Behavior, 7*(1), 53–68.

Watts-English, T., Fortson, B., Gibler, N., Hooper, S., & De Bellis, M. (2006). The psychobiology of maltreatment in childhood. *Journal of Social Sciences, 62*(4), 717–736.

Wegner, D., & Bargh, J. A. (1998). Control and automaticity in social life. In D. Gilbert, S. Fiske, & G. Lindzey (Eds.), *Handbook of social psychology (4/e)*. Boston: McGraw-Hill.

Williams, T., Connolly, J., Pepler, D., Craig, W., & Laporte, L. (2008). Risk models of dating aggression across different adolescent relationships: A developmental psychopathology approach. *Journal of Consulting and Clinical Psychology, 76*(4), 622–632.

Wittebrood, K., & Nieuwbeerta, P. (2000). Criminal victimization during one's life course: The effects of previous victimization and patterns of routine activities. *Journal of Research in Crime and Delinquency, 37*(1), 91–122.

Wolfe, D., Wekerle, C., Reitzel-Jaffe, D., & Lefebvre, L. (1998). Factors associated with abusive relationships among maltreated and non-maltreated youth. *Development and Psychopathology, 10*, 61–85.

Wolfgang, M., & Ferracuti, F. (1967). *The subculture of violence*. London: Tavistock.

Chapter 4
A Developmental Perspective on Interconnection

The within-person factors that we conceptualized as common causes of multiple forms of violence are proposed to be fairly stable over time as well as generalized across contexts. To understand the origins of these factors, in this chapter, we draw on developmental theory and research to explore how experiences in childhood and adolescence can give rise to the cognitive, emotional, biological, and behavioral processes described in Chap. 3. Exposure to abuse, maltreatment, and trauma is central to the development of all of these processes, but other kinds of experiences can play a formative role as well. We begin by describing normative and nonnormative developmental trajectories of aggressive behavior.

The Developmental Course of Aggression

Aggression is common in early childhood and can be observed across the peer, sibling, and parent relationships that comprise much of the world of young children. Physical aggression typically declines as children learn more socially acceptable ways to manage frustration and conflict and grow in their capacity to inhibit undesirable behavior (Coté et al. 2006). Socialization does not eliminate aggressive impulses; however, it moderates their expression and changes their form: as physically aggressive behavior diminishes during the school years, relational aggression may persist or even increase (Coté et al. 2007). Aggression decreases fastest against adults and persists the longest against peers, but in most cases it decreases to minimal levels by the time youth reach late adolescence or early adulthood.

However, there are subgroups of individuals whose behavior runs counter to these general developmental trends. Moffitt (1993) described two groups of youths who engage in high levels of antisocial and aggressive behavior during adolescence. "Adolescence-limited delinquents" exhibit a fairly low rate of aggression in childhood that rises early in adolescence and then returns to normative levels as they enter adulthood. Although they may engage in poly-perpetration for a short time, they tend not to commit the most serious offenses. The second group, "life

S. Hamby and J. Grych, *The Web of Violence*, SpringerBriefs in Sociology,
DOI: 10.1007/978-94-007-5596-3_4, © The Author(s) 2013

course persistent delinquents", demonstrates elevated levels of physical aggression in childhood that remain stable or increase over time. These individuals are at highest risk for perpetrating violence across relationships and to develop into repeat criminal perpetrators as adults (Woodward et al. 2002). Thus, they are the group most likely to be both repeat- and poly-perpetrators. The Diagnostic and Statistical Manual of Mental Disorders (American Psychiatric Association 2000) makes a similar distinction between conduct disorder that appears early in childhood versus adolescence. In addition to differences in age of onset, the early and late-onset groups have different developmental histories and prognoses for adult functioning. This two-group model does not fully account for all of the variability in aggressive trajectories—there are persistently aggressive adolescents who do not become violent adults and late-onset aggressive adolescents who continue to be violent in adulthood—but it has proven to be very useful for identifying pathways to chronic violent behavior.

As we discussed in Chap. 3, there are several common mechanisms that lead to increased risk of both perpetration and victimization of multiple types of violence. Because individual differences in aggression emerge early and remain fairly stable throughout life (Bushman and Huesmann 2010), the roots of repeat- and poly-perpetrator violence must be found in early childhood as well. Victimization experiences do not exhibit as much temporal stability as perpetration, but several pathways to polyvictimization and re-victimization have been identified that have their origins in childhood (Finkelhor et al. 2009a). Some of these pathways overlap with those described above, because life course delinquents often have been exposed to childhood victimization and maltreatment, and may be victims as well as perpetrators in later relationships. Consequently, understanding how early experiences affect children's development is critical for tracing the origins of the web of violence.

The Development of Risk Factors for Violence

The development of several individual characteristics can give rise to the co-occurrence of different forms of interpersonal violence. These include emotional and self-regulatory processes, which include physiological and neuropsychological factors, and cognitive constructs such as schemas, working models, and beliefs. Although each is conceptually distinct, these factors are interconnected, because they represent different facets of children's responses and efforts to adapt to challenging and stressful circumstances. Further, many children experience multiple risk situations, which heightens the interrelationships among forms of violence and compounds their effects on development.

Our emphasis on stressful life experiences does not imply that genetic contributions to violent behavior are unimportant. Indeed, aggression and antisociality show a strong genetic component (Raine 2008; Van Goozen et al. 2007), and there likely are genetic contributions to most if not all of the intrapersonal characteristics proposed to give rise to perpetration. For example, there appear to be biologically-based predispositions that make some individuals less sensitive to consequences and punishment (Raine 2008), which may lead to greater fearlessness or less concern for the impact of one's behavior on others. As this example suggests, it is likely that genes have a general effect on violent behavior and so may contribute to poly-perpetration. However, genes appear to influence behavior through complex interactions with experience; genetic predispositions can shape the way particular experiences affect children, and experiences can influence whether and how particular genes are expressed. For example, Caspi and his colleagues (2002) showed that children with one variant of the MAOI transporter gene exhibited higher levels of aggression as adults than those with a different variant of the MAOI gene, but only if they had been victims of maltreatment. Efforts to identify the specific genes implicated in violent perpetration, their mechanism of action, and the nature of their interactions with environmental factors are at an early stage and, as far as we are aware, genetic analyses of victimization have not been conducted. Consequently, we will focus on the environmental experiences that are most closely linked to violence—both perpetration and victimization–and its precursors.

The experiences that we describe below have effects on multiple risk processes. They can affect beliefs about the self and others, the justifiability of particular behaviors, the biological processes regulating arousal and affect, sensitivity to perceiving threat, the capacity to accurately read and express emotion, and the ability to inhibit impulses and manage goal-driven behavior. We organize these experiences roughly in chronological order, beginning in infancy. However, because some can occur at any point in childhood (e.g., maltreatment), the order in which they are presented is approximate.

Relationship with Caregivers

The origins of individuals' expectations for and beliefs about the self and others can be found in their earliest relationships. Attachment theory (Bowlby 1969) holds that interactions between caregivers and children early in life create a foundation for children's interpersonal relationships. Children develop expectations about the behavior of others and of their own worth through countless experiences in which caregivers respond (or fail to respond) to children's needs for comfort, safety, and nurturance. Working models of self and other are complementary: Children who experience consistently responsive and sensitive parenting develop views of others as trustworthy and caring and of themselves as worthy of care, whereas children who receive inconsistent or persistently neglectful or abusive care develop insecure working models in which important others are viewed as unpredictable, unavailable, disinterested, or hostile, and the self as unworthy of love. Working models are revised throughout life as a result of new relationship experiences, but because they guide expectations and behavior toward others, they tend to elicit congruent behavior that confirms the expectations, and thus tend to be self-perpetuating.

Caregiver-child interactions influence emotional development in myriad ways. Because infants' capacity for modulating their internal states is very limited, emotion regulation initially comes from external sources: parents calm and comfort their infants and later model strategies for reducing negative affect. Children then learn that distress is generally controllable and acquire specific control strategies. However, parents vary in attunement to children's emotional cues and ability to help them manage distress; children whose parents fail to soothe them, or worse, respond to their emotions punitively or dismissively, may become overwhelmed by negative affect. Failure to provide sensitive care increases children's stress, and has been linked to dysregulated HPA axis functioning, including elevated cortisol responses and slower returns to baseline (Albers et al. 2008; Haley and Stansbury 2003). In these circumstances, children not only fail to learn how to regulate strong emotions, they learn to fear and avoid them, and often struggle to inhibit angry and aggressive impulses later in life.

The research on caregiver-child relationships has important implications for understanding violence perpetration and victimization. Attachment security has been linked to both perpetration of violence and victimization in close relationships (e.g., Holtzworth-Munroe et al. 1997). Insecurely attached adults tend to be hypervigilant to signs of rejection or threats to the relationship, and thus ambiguous or benign behavior may be perceived in a way that triggers fear, anger, and aggression (e.g., Purdie and Downey 2000). Individuals with low self-worth who strongly desire intimate relationships may prioritize preserving a violent relationship over protecting themselves, and may perceive abuse as an acceptable cost of having a relationship. Those who are poorly attuned to their own emotions are at greater risk for both perpetration and victimization, because suppression or avoidance of emotional cues interferes with their ability to respond effectively to problems in their relationships.

How insecure attachment with a caregiver affects later aggressive behavior will be influenced by a variety of other factors. For example, the involvement of other adults who provide sensitive and responsive care provides a different kind of relationship model that can result in more flexible and positive views of both self and others. On the other hand, other kinds of adverse experiences in the family could compound the effects of insecure attachment. One of the most salient, which is often accompanied by disruptions in attachment, is maltreatment.

Child Maltreatment

Child maltreatment has pervasive effects on development. The sequelae of physical and sexual abuse and neglect include all of the common factors we described for interpersonal violence: social cognitive, affective, regulatory, and biological. First, maltreatment shapes the content of children's self-schemas. Children actively attempt to make sense of their experiences, and when caregivers are physically, sexually, or verbally abusive, they try to understand why it happened. Because of their limited capacity to decenter and take others' perspectives, young children may conclude that the abuse was caused by their own inadequacies. Abuse-related feelings of shame and anger have been found to predict abuse in teen dating relationships (Feiring et al. 2002). Abuse also influences children's beliefs and expectations about others in relationship. As we noted in Chap. 3, working models and schemas are very similar constructs (Bretherton and Munholland 1999), and maltreated children may develop the belief that abuse and aggression are a normative part of close relationships; these kinds of beliefs may lead to greater acceptance of abuse in adolescent and adult relationships and so greater risk of victimization and perpetration (Kinsfogel and Grych 2004). Although abuse and exposure to violence may have more obvious effects on children, the effects of parental neglect are at least as profound. Repeated experiences in which children's needs are ignored, dismissed, or punished send a pernicious message about their importance and value.

Maltreatment also can affect the development of emotion regulation. All forms of abuse produce significant emotional distress, which is magnified when the person expected to care for and comfort the child is the source of their distress. Toddlers and young children who have been victims of physical abuse show disruptions in emotional processing, including heightened sensitivity to anger, poorer recognition and expression of emotion, and difficulty modulating anger (Pollak et al. 2000; Shackman et al. 2007). Heightened sensitivity to anger is adaptive in environments where early detection of such cues might enable children to avoid abuse, but is likely to be maladaptive if it generalizes to nondangerous situations. Their heightened vigilance may lead children to perceive ambiguous cues as hostile and to become more physiologically and emotionally reactive to anger, which in turn are likely to increase the probability of aggressive responding.

In addition to affecting children's schemas, abusive experiences can undermine the physiological processes that underlie emotional and behavioral regulation. Accumulating evidence indicates that a range of stressful and traumatic events, including neglect, have similar effects on the biological stress response system, which includes the HPA axis, ANS, and immune responses (Maughan et al. 2007; Repetti et al. 2011; Saltzman et al. 2005). This integrated response increases physiological arousal and mobilizes behavioral responses to environmental threats; after the threat has passed, the system downregulates and these processes return to baseline levels. The allostatic load model holds that repeated exposure to stressful events dysregulates the human stress response system by keeping it in a heightened state of alert (Susman 2006). Over time, hyperarousal of this system depletes the physiological resources needed to respond adaptively to threat and undermines the capacity of individuals to mobilize effective reactions to new stressors (Repetti et al. 2011; Susman 2006). This model thus offers a common pathway through which early experiences of different forms of maltreatment affect later perpetration and victimization.

Family Conflict and Exposure to Other Forms of Aggression

There are aspects of family functioning in addition to parent–child attachment and abuse that also predict violence in interpersonal relationships. In particular, witnessing interparental aggression and aggressive sibling relationships have been linked to higher rates of violence perpetration and victimization in peer and romantic relationships (e.g., Bank et al. 2004; Graham-Bermann et al. 1994; Hamby et al. 2012; Kinsfogel and Grych 2004; Marcus et al. 2001). These experiences appear to affect relationship functioning in much the same way as described for maltreatment. Exposure to anger and aggression between caregivers and with siblings can shape the development of beliefs and expectations about the self and others in close relationships and reinforce the use of aggression. These experiences thus may contribute to the development of interpersonal schemas in which hostility, rejection, and the threat of violence figure prominently. Children with such schemas enter into new situations and relationships with heightened sensitivity to threat, and hypervigilant to signs of rejection, anger, or aggression. Their responses to perceived provocation could vary, however. Children who witness interpersonal aggression may learn both roles in aggressor-victim relationships, and thus they could exhibit a withdrawn or submissive orientation in which they attempt to avoid conflict or mistreatment, or an aggressive, dominant orientation in which they prevent victimization by striking first.

Exposure to conflict and aggression in and outside of the family also have been linked to the functioning of the HPA axis and other indicators of the biological stress response (Davies et al. 2007; Saltzman et al. 2005). Early childhood experiences may be particularly influential, because brain development is particularly vulnerable to environmental stress (Dawson et al. 2000; Susman 2006). Thus, children living in dangerous neighborhoods who witness crime and violence may experience chronically elevated stress responses, and poverty may compromise health through biological processes that are affected by stress (e.g., immune functioning; Shirtcliff et al. 2009).

Peer Relationships

Although family experiences have a profound effect on children's development, peers present a second major relationship context for establishing interpersonal patterns. When they enter the school or preschool setting, children face a new social world that presents both opportunities and challenges. In contrast to the family, where children's roles are constrained by age and birth order, the peer context offers a field of similarly sized, similarly aged individuals with no pre-established social structure. This affords the potential to create more egalitarian and reciprocal relationships and to develop a host of interpersonal skills relevant to working and playing collaboratively, negotiating differences, and establishing friendships. However, social hierarchies typically emerge, and bullying becomes part of the landscape as some children use aggression to exert power over peers and attain status in the peer group.

Some bullying is overt and physical, especially earlier in childhood, but it also can involve verbal or relational behavior in which injury is more likely to be psychological than physical: public humiliation, denigration, or social exclusion. Bullying also can take the form of sexual and gender-based harassment, when the demand to fit into gender role expectations can lead to boys being teased and derided for being insufficiently masculine and girls becoming the target of sexual comments, jokes, and unwanted touching (Chiodo et al. 2009; Wolfe et al. 2009). Bullying generally peaks in middle school and declines over the course of high school, and tends to be more common when children transition into new social arenas.

Depending on how narrowly bullying is defined and the source of data (self, peers, or teachers), research indicates that as many as 25–35 % of youths have experienced some bullying (Finkelhor et al. 2009). For many, engaging in or being the target of peer aggression is infrequent or time limited; however, there are some who exhibit a consistent pattern of bullying, victimization, or both (Pepler et al. 2008; Sourander et al. 2000). In general, victims of bullying and peer aggression tend to be withdrawn, submissive, and less popular than youths who are not bullied; they may be viewed as "easy targets" who will not fight back or seek help from teachers or other authorities (e.g., Card 2011, Espelage and Holt 2001). Bullies are a heterogeneous group with different developmental trajectories and motives for aggression (e.g., Pepler et al. 2008). Some of these youths engage in bullying as a way to gain status in the peer group, and it often diminishes once their position is established. Other bullies exhibit continuously high levels of aggression that reflects a general tendency to engage in antisocial and delinquent behavior, and often occurs in the context of more pervasive social and academic problems. The perpetrator-victim group tends to exhibit the poorest psychological adjustment (Espelage and Holt 2007; Pope and Bierman 1999; Schwartz 2000). They demonstrate poor affect and behavior regulation, impulsivity, poor academic performance, low levels of prosocial behavior, and elevated rates of anxiety and depression. These unskilled, unpopular children experience more social rejection from peers, perhaps because they overreact to common situations such as teasing, and tend to strike out aggressively against others.

Both bullying and being bullied can affect the cognitive, emotional, and physiological processes linked to violence in adulthood. Experiences with peers contribute to the development and differentiation of interpersonal schemas that originated earlier in childhood. Youths who are bullied may develop representations of others as aggressive, untrustworthy, and uncaring, and view themselves as unlikable and ineffectual. Bullies may have similar conceptions of peer relationships, but also believe that aggression is a justifiable and effective way to gain status and self-worth. Because aggressive and delinquent youths tend to affiliate, these attitudes are likely to be reinforced by like-minded friends who support and encourage hostile views and aggressive behavior (Capaldi et al. 2001; Dishion et al. 1995). For both aggressors and victims, power may become a highly salient aspect of interpersonal relationships, and the motivation to avoid becoming a victim may drive many of their interactions with peers. As noted above, victims (including those who also bully) experience higher levels of anxiety and depression, which may further their withdrawal and isolation. They also exhibit greater emotional reactivity, and continued victimization is likely to amplify dysregulation of the stress response system.

Links Between Family and Peer Contexts

Although the peer context provides new opportunities for healthy relationships, children are not equally prepared to take advantage of these opportunities. They enter the world of peer relations with predispositions shaped by their experiences in family, and are more or less equipped to engage in prosocial, reciprocal relationships, to assert themselves in constructive ways, and to manage their impulses and feelings. Children who bully or are bullied tend to report more exposure to a range of family risk factors, including maltreatment, harsh discipline, exposure to intimate partner violence, and conflictual parent–child relationships (Finkelhor et al. 2009; Pepler et al. 2008). For example, maltreatment may lead to anxious or withdrawn behavior that makes children attractive targets to bullies. A recent 25-year longitudinal study documented connections between family and peer relationships over three generations, showing that exposure to intimate partner violence in childhood predicted later peer victimization, and the most severe IPV exposure predicted both bullying and victimization, even after controlling for internalizing and externalizing problems (Knous-Westfall, Ehrensaft, MacDonell, and Cohen, 2012).

A 7-year longitudinal study that followed 800 children from elementary school through high school illustrates these connections over time and across contexts (Pepler et al. 2008). Pepler and colleagues identified four trajectories of bullying behavior: youths who engaged in little or no bullying (42 %); youths who exhibited moderate levels of bullying in elementary school that diminished over time (13 %); youths who consistently engaged in moderate levels of bullying (35 %); and youths who exhibited high levels of bullying that increased from elementary through high school (10 %). The latter two groups differed significantly from the first two on all of the risk factors assessed, including individual (moral disengagement), family (parental monitoring and closeness, parent–child conflict), and peer (association with aggressive peers, susceptibility to peer influence, conflict with peers) characteristics. The persistent bullies closely resemble life course persistent delinquents in that they exhibited early signs of aggression, little regard for the feelings or welfare of others, and troubled family and peer relationships. The group that engaged in bullying in elementary school but desisted over time differed from the group that never engaged in bullying on only one risk factor: susceptibility to peer influences. This group appears to consist of youths who have basically good relationships and engage in bullying as a way to establish social status early in elementary school. Once they attain status, they cease bullying, and have the interpersonal skills to maintain their status through more prosocial means.

This research supports the idea that the cognitive, affective, behavioral, and biological sequelae of stressful and abusive experiences in the family influence children's capacity to engage in healthy peer relationships. Children who enter the peer arena with poor emotional and behavioral regulation will have more difficulty responding to frustration and normative levels of teasing and rough play. Those with interpersonal schemas in which aggression, threat, and mistrust are salient are at high risk to perpetuate the maladaptive relationship patterns initiated in the family. Although the content of these schemas may be represented in explicit beliefs about the use of aggression, the presence of nonconscious, automatic thoughts that arise instantaneously in social interactions are likely to be powerful influences on behavior as well, particularly for children who struggle to control their emotional and behavioral reactions.

Romantic Relationships in Adolescence

A third major interpersonal context emerges in adolescence when many youths begin to engage in romantic and sexual relationships. Establishing intimate relationships is viewed as a key developmental task of adolescence (Masten and Coatsworth 1998) that offers opportunities to develop greater emotional intimacy and express sexual needs and feelings in the context of a close relationship. However, these relationships also present a new source of potential violence exposure (Malik et al. 1997; Wolitzky-Taylor et al. 2008). Although estimates have ranged as high as 50 %, the largest and most representative US samples indicate that 6–12 % of adolescents report that a boyfriend or girlfriend has hit, slapped, or physically hurt them (CDC 2012; Halpern et al. 2001; Hamby et al. 2012). Psychological abuse is at least twice as common in this age group (Halpern et al. 2001; Jouriles et al. 2009). The physical aggression reported by adolescents often appears to be mild, and sometimes may be intended to be playful or flirtatious (Capaldi and Gorman-Smith 2003; Jouriles et al. 2009). Nonetheless, a substantial portion of it is quite serious, with more than a one-third of victimized girls (36 %) and 12 % of victimized boys reporting injury from teen dating violence in recent US data (Hamby et al. 2012).

Perpetration and victimization of teen physical and psychological dating violence tend to be highly correlated, leading many to conclude that aggression in these relationships is mutual or reciprocal, and unrelated to gender. However, reliance on cross-sectional research designs and retrospective reports of aggression covering lengthy time periods (often a year) make it impossible to draw conclusions about the dynamics of dating aggression. As discussed in Chap. 2, definitions of perpetrator-victim status tend to be more simplistic in the teen dating violence literature than in other areas. There has been little attention to the differences between interactions in which two people engage equally in physical aggression and interactions in which one partner frequently perpetrates aggression and the other fights back once or rarely. In both cases, each partner could be considered a perpetrator and a victim, but those designations would obscure potentially important differences between the relationships. As we discuss further in Chap. 5, more nuanced attention to perpetrator-victim patterns is needed to better understand this dynamic.

The extent to which dating violence represents a stable pattern of behavior in adolescence also is unclear. Continuity in aggression toward dating partners in adolescence would suggest that adult intimate partner violence has its roots—and perhaps its prevention—in these early romantic relationships. Early studies suggested considerable continuity in aggression toward romantic partners, especially for males (Cano et al. 1998; Chase et al. 1998; O'Leary and Slep 2003), but the cross-sectional, retrospective nature of these studies cloud the interpretation of the results. More recent studies suggest that aggression toward dating partners is at best moderately stable. For example, Williams and colleagues (2008) assessed high school students aged 14–19 at two time points, 1 year apart. They included only youths who were involved with different partners at the two time points (86 % of the sample), and found that 13 % reported engaging in physical aggression in both relationships, whereas 32 % indicated that aggression occurred in only one relationship; the remaining participants (55 %) did not report any aggression. Correlations between the frequency of engaging in and being the target of aggressive behavior at the two time points ranged from 0.34 to 0.44 (for similar results, see Wolfe et al. 2004).

It may be that there are meaningful subgroups of youths involved in dating aggression that parallel those found for bullying. That is, some repeat perpetrators may consistently exhibit aggression over time and across partners, whereas the aggressive behavior of others may be specific to particular relationships. There is very little research on this question, but one study conducted with young adults suggests that youths' developmental histories do predict their behavior toward dating partners. Woodward et al. (2002) found that 21-year-olds exhibited higher levels of perpetration toward current romantic partners if they reported an onset of antisocial behavior in childhood than if their antisocial behavior began in adolescence. This finding held up after accounting for several factors associated with early onset conduct disorder. This study adds to the accumulating evidence that individuals who exhibit aggressive and antisocial behavior early in life are at high risk to continue to perpetrate violence in multiple relationship contexts over the lifespan.

Work by Williams and her colleagues (2008) also indicated that the causes of relationship violence are complex and may differ across individuals. They reported that adolescents' attitudes about the justifiability of aggression moderated the association between peer and dating aggression: For youths who perceived violence as justifiable, their level of aggression toward peers was a significant predictor of dating aggression; for those who were low in aggressive attitudes, only the level of conflict in the dating relationship predicting dating aggression. These findings suggest that youths with particular individual characteristics (in this case, explicit beliefs about aggression) may exhibit stability in their aggression across romantic relationships, whereas for others dating violence primarily is a product of relationship factors. They also highlight the importance of extending the usual focus on individual characteristics to incorporate the nature of the interaction that develops between partners in understanding violence in romantic relationships.

Links Among Peer, Dating, and Family Relationships

Romantic relationships can be conceptualized as a bridge between adolescent friendships and adult intimate relationships; consequently, the quality of youths' peer relationships is expected to have implications for their romantic relationships. Indeed, victims of teen dating violence report higher levels of a wide variety of peer victimizations, including bullying (Espelage and Holt 2007. Teens who engage in peer aggression also are more likely to perpetrate dating violence (Connolly et al. 2000; Kim and Capaldi 2004). Other research has found that both perpetration and victimization in peer relationships were related to both perpetration and victimization in dating relationships (Williams et al. 2008), and so the lines between the perpetrator or victim role across the two relationships may not be firm.

The connections across the two relationship contexts also may reflect broader processes that go beyond aggressive behavior. The occurrence of violence may be one indicator of recurrent difficulties in establishing and maintaining healthy relationships. For example, Williams and her colleagues (2008) found that in addition to reporting more dating aggression, youths who bullied their peers also became involved in dating earlier and had more negative views of relationships with both friends and dating partners, rating them as less intimate, affectionate, equitable, and stable than did youths who were not involved in bullying. Thus, many of the same factors that undermine same-sex friendships are likely to affect romantic relationships; although some may arise in adolescence, others have their origins in family relationships. In fact, many of the same family factors that predict peer aggression (e.g., maltreatment, exposure to intimate partner violence) also predict dating violence (Kinsfogel and Grych 2004; Wolfe et al. 1998), most likely through the same mechanisms. For example, Wolfe et al. (1998) found that interpersonal hostility mediated the association between child maltreatment and dating aggression for girls and was an independent predictor for boys, and Kinsfogel and Grych (2004) reported that anger regulation mediated the link between interparental aggression and dating aggression for boys and girls.

Attachment security also has been linked to aggression in adolescent dating relationships (Feiring et al. 2002; Levandosky et al. 2002). Rather than directly predicting aggression; however, it appears to moderate the relationship between prior experiences with exposure to aggression and aggression in adolescent dating relationships. Grych and Kinsfogel (2010) found a stronger relationship between exposure to family aggression and engaging in physical aggression toward a dating partner among boys high in attachment anxiety compared to those with more secure attachment. For girls, avoidance moderated the association between exposure to family aggression and aggression in dating relationships (also see Wekerle and Wolfe 1998). Further, attachment quality also interacted with adolescents' attitudes about aggression and ability to regulate anger in predicting dating aggression. For individuals who perceive aggression to be justifiable in close relationships, the fear that their partner is not committed to the relationship or wants to end it may lead them to engage in coercive or abusive behavior in an effort to maintain the relationship. Aggression also may occur because anxious boys with poor regulatory abilities become angry when they perceive the threat of rejection; their fear of losing the relationship may further increase their emotional arousal beyond a point where they can effectively manage it. These findings thus suggest that secure working models about romantic relationships can attenuate the impact of cognitive and emotional processes on aggressive behavior.

Relationship experiences in adolescence have been posited to influence how one relates to romantic partners in adulthood (O'Leary, Malone, and Tyree, 1994; Wolfe et al. 2004). Unfortunately, very little is known about how relationship experiences during early adolescence influence relationship functioning over the course of adolescence (let alone from adolescence to adulthood).

Conclusion

The theory and research described in this chapter provide a developmental perspective for understanding continuity in violence over time and across relationship contexts. This work indicates that the roots of poly-perpetration and poly-victimization can be found early in childhood and traced through family, peer, and romantic relationships as they unfold and expand through adolescence and into adulthood. Experiences with caregivers and interactions in the family more broadly shape children's beliefs about the self and others in relationships, their capacity to regulate affect, and their behavioral repertoire. Exposure to adverse events, including violence and maltreatment, also disrupt biological processes that underlie the human stress response, and lead to emotional and behavioral dysregulation that impair individuals' capacity to respond adaptively to threatening situations. The processes that give rise to aggressive behavior and increase vulnerability to victimization in turn are reinforced by interactions with others throughout childhood and adolescence. Children who become dysregulated under stress, have difficulty managing anger, perceive threat and hostility in ambiguous situations, and view violence as justifiable are more likely to have conflictual and coercive interactions with family members, peers, and romantic partners. The discord and rejection that can result confirms or exacerbates the processes that lead to aggressive behavior, resulting in a transactional, cascading cycle that becomes increasingly difficult to change over time. This cycle also blurs the distinction between person and situation factors, because individuals with greater predispositions to engage in violence tend to select into and create situations in which threat and provocation are more likely to occur.

Although the way that various relationships build on and reflect each other contributes to interlinkages among violence forms, it is worth mentioning again that these patterns are not inevitabilities. Although family processes may orient children toward bullying or being bullied, perpetrating against or being victimized by dating partners, it is also possible for healthy relationships with peers, dating partners, or influential adults to deflect this trajectory. Children without prior vulnerabilities may also have peer or dating experiences that result in violence occurring in their relationships. Nonetheless, these intersecting trajectories and influences highlight areas that might benefit from further attention. In the next chapter, we address how recognizing the interconnections among different forms of violence over the lifespan can enhance research investigating the causes and consequences of interpersonal violence.

References

Albers, E., Riksen-Walraven, J., Sweep, F., & Weerth, C. (2008). Maternal behavior predicts infant cortisol recovery from a mild everyday stressor. *Journal of Child Psychology and Psychiatry, 49*, 97–103.

American Psychiatric Association. (2000). *Diagnostic and statistical manual of mental disorders DSM-IV TR Fourth edition (Text revision)*. Washington: Author.

Bank, L., Burraston, B., & Snyder, J. (2004). Sibling conflict and ineffective parenting as predictors of adolescent boys' antisocial behavior and peer difficulties: Additive and interactional effects. *Journal of Research on Adolescence, 14*, 99–125.

Bowlby, J. (1969). *Attachment and loss: Vol. 1. attachment*. London: Hogarth.

Bretherton, I., & Munholland, K. (1999). Internal working models in attachment: A construct revisited. In J. Cassidy & P. Shaver (Eds.), *Handbook of attachment: Theory, research and clinical application* (pp. 89–111). New York: Guilford.

Bushman, B. J., & Huesmann, L. (2010). Aggression. In S. T. Fiske, D. T. Gilbert, & G. Lindzey (Eds.), *Handbook of social psychology* (5th ed., pp. 833–863). New York: John Wiley & Sons.

Cano, A., Avery-Leaf, S., Cascardi, M., & O'Leary, K. D. (1998). Dating violence in two high schools: Discriminating variables. *Journal of Primary Prevention, 18*, 431–446.

Capaldi, D., & Gorman-Smith, D. (2003). The development of aggression in young male/female couples. In P. Florsheim (Ed.), *Adolescent romantic relations and sexual behavior: Theory, research and practical implications* (pp. 243–278). Mahwah: Lawrence Erlbaum Associates.

Capaldi, D., Dishion, T., Stoolmiller, M., & Yoerger, K. (2001). Aggression toward female partners by at-risk young men: The contribution of male adolescent friendships. *Developmental Psychology, 37*, 61–73.

Card, N. (2011). Toward a relationship perspective on aggression among schoolchildren: Integrating social cognitive and interdependence theories. *Psychology of Violence, 1*(3), 188–201.

CDC. (2012). Youth risk behavior surveillance: United States, 2011. *Morbidity and Mortality Weekly Reports, 61*(4), 1–162.

Chase, K., Treboux, D., O'Leary, K. D., & Strassberg, Z. (1998). Specificity of dating aggression and its justification among high-risk adolescents. *Journal of Abnormal Child Psychology, 26*(6), 467–473.

Chiodo, D., Wolfe, D., Crooks, C., Hughes, R., & Jaffe, P. (2009). Impact of sexual harassment victimization by peers on subsequent adolescent victimization and adjustment: A longitudinal study. *Journal of Adolescent Health, 45*, 246–252.

Connolly, J., Pepler, D., Craig, W., & Taradash, A. (2000). Dating experiences of bullies in early adolescence. *Child Maltreatment, 5*, 299–310.

Coté, S., Vaillancourt, T., LeBlanc, J., Nagin, D., & Tremblay, R. (2006). The development of physical aggression from toddlerhood to pre-adolescence: A nationwide longitudinal study of Canadian children. *Journal of Abnormal Child Psychology, 34*, 71–85.

Coté, S., Vaillancourt, T., Barker, E., Nagin, D., & Tremblay, R. (2007). The joint development of physical and indirect aggression: Predictors of continuity and change during childhood. *Development and Psychopathology, 19*, 37–55.

Davies, P., Sturge-Apple, M., Cicchetti, D., & Cummings, E. (2007). The role of child adreno-cortical functioning in pathways between forms of interparental conflict and child maladjust-ment. *Developmental Psychology, 43*, 918–930.

Dawson, G., Ashman, S., & Carver, L. (2000). The role of early experience in shaping behav-ioral and brain development and its implications for social policy. *Development and Psychopathology, 12*, 695–712.

Dishion, T., Andrews, D., & Crosby, L. (1995). Antisocial boys and their friends in early ado-lescence: Relationship characteristics, quality, and interactional process. *Child Development, 66*, 139–151.

Espelage, D. L., & Holt, M. K. (2001). Bullying and victimization during early adolescence. *Journal of Emotional Abuse, 2*(2-3), 123–142. doi: 10.1300/J135v02n02_08

Espelage, D., & Holt, M. (2007). Dating violence and sexual harassment across the bully-victim con-tinuum among middle and high school students. *Journal of Youth and Adolescence, 36*, 799–811.

Feiring, C., Deblinger, E., Hoch-Espada, A., & Haworth, T. (2002). Romantic relationship aggression and attitudes in high school students: The role of gender, grade, and attachment and emotional styles. *Journal of Youth and Adolescence, 31*(5), 373–385.

Finkelhor, D., Ormrod, R., Turner, H., & Holt, M. (2009a). Pathways to poly-victimization. *Child Maltreatment, 14*(4), 316–329.

Finkelhor, D., Turner, H., Ormrod, R., & Hamby, S. (2009b). Violence, abuse and crime exposure in a national sample of children and youth. *Pediatrics, 124*, 1411–1423.

Graham-Bermann, S., Cutler, S., Litzenberger, B., & Schwartz, W. (1994). Perceived conflict and violence in childhood sibling relationships and later emotional adjustment. *Journal of Family Psychology, 8*, 85–97.

Grych, J. H., & Kinsfogel, K. (2010). Exploring the role of attachment style in the rela-tion between family aggression and abuse in adolescent dating relationships. *Journal of Aggression, Maltreatment, and Trauma, 19*, 624–664.

Haley, D., & Stansbury, K. (2003). Infant stress and parent responsiveness: Regulation of physi-ology and behavior during still-face and reunion. *Child Development, 74*(5), 1534–1546.

Halpern, C., Oslak, S., Young, M., Martin, S., & Kupper, L. (2001). Partner violence among ado-lescents in opposite-sex romantic relationships: Findings from the National Longitudinal Study of Adolescent Health. *American Journal of Public Health, 91*(10), 1679–1685.

Hamby, S., Finkelhor, D., & Turner, H. (2012). Teen dating violence: Co-occurrence with other victimizations in the National Survey of Children's Exposure to Violence (NatSCEV). *Psychology of Violence, 2*(2), 111–124. doi:10.1037/a0027191.

Holtzworth-Munroe, A., Stuart, G., & Hutchinson, G. (1997). Violent versus nonviolent hus-bands: Differences in attachment patterns, dependency, and jealousy. *Journal of Family Psychology, 11*, 314–331.

Jouriles, E., Garrido, E., McDonald, R., & Rosenfield, D. (2009). Psychological and physical aggression in adolescent romantic relationships: Links to psychological distress. *Child Abuse and Neglect, 33*, 451–460.

Kim, H., & Capaldi, D. (2004). The association of antisocial behavior and depressive symp-toms between partners and risk for aggression in romantic relationships. *Journal of Family Psychology, 18*, 82–96.

Kinsfogel, K., & Grych, J. H. (2004). Interparental conflict and adolescent dating relationships: Integrating cognitive, emotional, and peer influences. *Journal of Family Psychology, 18*, 505–515.

Knous-Westfall, H., Ehrensaft, M., Watson MacDonell, K., & Cohen, P. (2012). Parental inti-mate partner violence, parenting practices, and adolescent peer bullying: A prospective study. *Journal of Child & Family Studies, 21*(5), 754–766. doi: 10.1007/s10826-011-9528-2

Levandosky, A., Huth-Bocks, A., & Semel, M. (2002). Adolescent peer relationships and men-tal health functioning in families with domestic violence. *Journal of Clinical Child and Adolescent Psychology, 31*, 206–218.

Malik, S., Sorenson, S., & Aneshensel, C. (1997). Community and dating violence among ado-lescents: Perpetration and victimization. *Journal of Adolescent Health, 21*, 291–302.

Marcus, N., Lindahl, K., & Malik, N. (2001). Interparental conflict, children's social cognitions, and child aggression: A test of a mediational model. *Journal of Family Psychology, 15,* 315–333.

Masten, A., & Coatsworth, J. (1998). The development of competence in favorable and unfavorable environments: Lessons from research on successful children. *American Psychologist, 53,* 205–220.

Maughan, A., Cicchetti, D., Toth, S., & Rogosch, F. (2007). Early-occurring maternal depression and maternal negativity in predicting young children's emotion regulation and socioemotional difficulties. *Journal of Abnormal Child Psychology, 35,* 685–703.

Moffitt, T. E. (1993). Adolescence-limited and life-course-persistent antisocial behavior: A developmental taxonomy. *Psychological Review, 100*(4), 674–701.

O'Leary, K. D., Malone, J., & Tyree, A. (1994). Physical aggression in early marriage: Prerelationship and relationship effects. *Journal of Consulting and Clinical Psychology, 62*(3), 594–602. doi: 10.1037/0022-006x.62.3.594

O'Leary, K. D., & Slep, A. M. S. (2003). A dyadic longitudinal model of adolescent dating aggression. *Journal of Clinical Child and Adolescent Psychology, 32*(3), 314–327.

Pepler, D., Jiang, D., Craig, W., & Connolly, J. (2008). Developmental trajectories of bullying and associated factors. *Child Development, 79,* 325–338.

Pollak, S., Cicchetti, D., Hornung, K., & Reed, A. (2000). Recognizing emotions in faces: Developmental effects of child abuse and neglect. *Developmental Psychology, 36,* 679–688.

Pope, A., & Bierman, K. (1999). Predicting adolescent peer problems and antisocial activities: The relative roles of aggression and dysregulation. *Developmental Psychology, 35,* 335–346.

Purdie, V., & Downey, G. (2000). Rejection sensitivity and adolescent girls' vulnerability to relationship-centered difficulties. *Child Maltreatment, 5,* 338–349.

Raine, A. (2008). From genes to brain to antisocial behavior. *Current Directions in Psychological Science, 17,* 323–328.

Repetti, R., Robles, T., & Reynolds, B. (2011). Allostatic processes in the family. *Development and Psychopathology, 23,* 921–938.

Saltzman, K., Holden, G., & Holahan, C. (2005). The psychobiology of children exposed to marital violence. *Journal of Clinical Child and Adolescent Psychology, 34,* 129–139.

Schwartz, D. (2000). Subtypes of victims and aggressors in children's peer groups. *Journal of Abnormal Child Psychology, 28,* 181–192.

Shackman, J., Shackman, A., & Pollak, S. (2007). Physical abuse amplifies attention to threat and increases anxiety in children. *Emotion, 7,* 838–852.

Shirtcliff, E. A., Coe, C. L., & Pollak, S. D. (2009). Early childhood stress is associated with elevated antibody levels to herpes simplex virus type 1. *Proceedings of the National Academy of Sciences, 106*(8), 2963–2967. doi: 10.1073/pnas.0806660106

Sourander, A., Helstela, L., Heleinus, H., & Piha, J. (2000). Persistence of bullying from childhood to adolescence—a longitudinal 8 year follow-up study. *Child Abuse and Neglect, 24,* 873–881.

Susman, E. (2006). Psychobiology of persistent antisocial behavior: Stress, early vulnerabilities and the attenuation hypothesis. *Neuroscience and Biobehavioral Reviews, 30,* 376–389.

Van Goozen, S., Fairchild, G., Snoek, H., & Harold, G. (2007). The evidence for a neurobiological model of childhood antisocial behavior. *Psychological Bulletin, 133,* 149–182.

Wekerle, C., & Wolfe, D. A. (1998). The role of child maltreatment and attachment style in adolescent relationship violence. *Development and Psychopathology, 10*(3), 571–586.

Williams, T., Connolly, J., Pepler, D., Craig, W., & Laporte, L. (2008). Risk models of dating aggression across different adolescent relationships: A developmental psychopathology approach. *Journal of Consulting and Clinical Psychology, 76*(4), 622–632.

Wolfe, D., Wekerle, C., Reitzel-Jaffe, D., & Lefebvre, L. (1998). Factors associated with abusive relationships among maltreated and non-maltreated youth. *Development and Psychopathology, 10,* 61–85.

Wolfe, D., Wekerle, C., Scott, K., Straatman, A., & Grasley, C. (2004). Predicting abuse in adolescent dating relationships over 1 year: The role of child maltreatment and trauma. *Journal of Abnormal Psychology, 113,* 406–415.

Wolfe, D., Crooks, C., Jaffe, P. G., Chiodo, D., Hughes, R., Ellis, W., et al. (2009). A school-based program to prevent adolescent dating violence. *Archives of Pediatric and Adolescent Medicine, 163*(8), 692–699.

Wolitzky-Taylor, K., Ruggiero, K. J., Danielson, C., Resnick, H., Hanson, R., Smith, D., et al. (2008). Prevalence and correlates of dating violence in a national sample of adolescents. *Journal of the American Academy of Child and Adolescent Psychiatry, 47*(7), 755–762.

Woodward, L., Fergusson, D., & Horwood, L. (2002). Romantic relationships of young people with childhood and adolescent onset antisocial behavior problems. *Journal of Abnormal Child Psychology, 30*(3), 231–243.

Chapter 5
Implications for Research: Toward a More Comprehensive Understanding of Interpersonal Violence

Recognition of the interconnections among different forms of interpersonal violence has critical implications for conducting research that can produce valid conclusions about the causes and consequences of abuse, maltreatment, and trauma. Although we are not suggesting that every study thoroughly assess every form of violence, nor that every researcher become expert in all types of abuse and maltreatment, conceptualizing them as the product of interrelated risk processes and intertwined developmental trajectories should change "business as usual" in which particular forms of violence are studied in isolation, and help to spur a more integrative approach to research that will take our understanding of violence to a new level.

An emphasis on co-occurrence generates new questions that do not arise from a singular focus on one type of violence. For example, does the effect of a particular kind of violence differ depending on what other kinds have been experienced? Do the additive or interactive effects depend on the particular combination of violence experienced, or features of the violence, such as the number of different settings, number of different perpetrators, or severity of the incidents? Why do some individuals engage in multiple forms of violence, whereas others are aggressive only in certain relationships contexts? Expanding violence research to incorporate multiple interrelated forms of violence increases the complexity of the task of studying them, and requires new conceptual frameworks for organizing and guiding empirical investigation. In this chapter we discuss the theoretical and methodological issues that arise from adopting a co-occurrence framework and offer ideas for conducting research that provides a more comprehensive and integrative understanding of interpersonal violence.

Developing Models of Interconnection for Interpersonal Violence

Existing theories for understanding violence tend to focus either on the general propensity to engage in aggressive or violent behavior (i.e., who is more or less likely to be violent) or the occurrence of violence in a particular context (i.e., what

S. Hamby and J. Grych, *The Web of Violence*, SpringerBriefs in Sociology, DOI: 10.1007/978-94-007-5596-3_5, © The Author(s) 2013

leads to bullying or intimate partner violence). Explaining the interconnections across forms of violence involves integrating these approaches and accounting for two sources of variability: variability across contexts and variability across people. The models that evolve from this approach necessarily will be developmental in nature in order to understand how experiences with a particular type of violence at one point in time increase (or decrease) the likelihood of others occurring later.

Although virtually all forms of interpersonal violence are associated with virtually all other forms, the magnitude of these associations vary (see Chap. 2 for details). Some forms, such as intimate partner violence and child maltreatment, show moderate to large associations, whereas others are small. A model of the interconnections among types of violence needs to explain why some types are more closely related than others. Different relationship contexts present impelling, inhibiting, and instigating forces that make particular kinds of situations more or less similar to each other, but situational factors are not sufficient to explain the degree of co-occurrence of different forms of violence. There also are individual differences in the generality of violent behavior: some people tend to be aggressive in a wide variety of situations, whereas others are violent only in specific contexts. For example, some men who engage in intimate partner violence are aggressive only toward their partners, whereas others exhibit aggression in a broad range of relationships (e.g., Holtzworth-Monroe and Stuart 1994). Thus, in addition to intrapersonal and situational factors that generally increase or decrease the likelihood of violent behavior, there likely are person-by-situation interactions in which particular individual characteristics are "triggered" by particular situational characteristics. Understanding the patterns of co-occurrence that exist over time and across contexts requires theoretical models that incorporate all three sources of variations (individual, situational, and their interaction) and describe how multiple types of interpersonal violence relate to each other and to individuals' mental and physical health. Such integrative models would have the additional benefit of encouraging researchers with different areas of expertise to conceptualize interpersonal violence in similar terms and so enhance the flow of information across disciplines and subdisciplines.

Progress in understanding the co-occurrence of violence does not depend solely on developing such broad, unifying theories, however. There are a variety of ways to incorporate awareness of the interconnections among types of violence that are smaller in scope. Nearly any effort to consider how particular forms of violence may be related to other forms can contribute to breaking down disciplinary silos and building a more integrated approach to understanding violence. Perhaps the most immediate way to advance theoretical progress is to expand existing models that focus on a particular type of violence by incorporating other types as risk factors, causes, consequences, or covarying outcomes. There have been a number of such efforts, including work that addresses different forms of family violence (Grych and Kinsfogel 2010; Hamby et al. 2010) and the links between bullying and dating violence (Rothman et al. 2010). Whether the scope of new or newly modified models is large or small, they will need to address three issues: the role of common and specific factors, developmental processes, and the relation between perpetration and victimization.

The Roles of Common and Specific Factors

In the course of systematically investigating risk and causal processes that are common to multiple types of violence, it is also important to identify factors that are unique to particular types. In Chap. 3, we discussed a set of constructs that may function as causal, risk, and vulnerability factors across most types of violence, and also described factors that may be unique to particular forms. For example, the biological stress response and the concept of allostatic load (Repetti et al. 2011) offer mechanisms for understanding how experiences with different types of violence may give rise to both perpetration and victimization of diverse forms of violence. Similarly, focusing on how exposure to different forms of violence may affect youths' representations of self or others may offer insight into connections between abusive or neglectful caregiving experiences and aggression toward or from peers in adolescence. Others processes may be more specific to particular contexts. For example, attachment needs are strongly elicited in romantic relationships and so may be especially pertinent for explaining perpetration and victimization in adolescent and adult intimate relationships. There may be other cognitive processes that are unique to certain relationship or situational contexts (e.g., parent–child relationship, intimate partner).

There are also existing models that can guide empirical research. Bushman and Anderson's General Aggression Model (Anderson and Bushman 2002) is one of the few theoretical frameworks intended to explain a wide range of aggressive and violent behavior. It identifies general classes of constructs proposed to be relevant to all forms of perpetration, though it does not address which may be more or less relevant for particular forms. The I^3 model developed by Finkel and his colleagues (Finkel 2008; Finkel et al. 2009) organizes an array of individual and situational factors according to their function in the genesis of violent behavior. Although their analysis focused on intimate partner violence, applying the concepts of impelling and inhibiting forces and instigating triggers to other forms of perpetration could facilitate the identification of constructs that are common (and unique) across contexts.

Another way of expanding on existing work would be to apply constructs studied in one subfield of violence research to other forms. For example, automatic cognitions are well studied in serious offenders (Gilbert and Daffern 2010) and are even beginning to be addressed in some interventions for serious offenders (Ciardha and Gannon 2011; Gannon et al. 2007), but have only recently been examined in other types of violence (see Jouriles et al. 2011 for an example of an extension to TDV). Using similar methods to assess these constructs will further enhance the comparability of results across studies. Relatedly, in documenting the effects of different forms of violence, assessing similar sets of outcomes will help to illuminate which sequelae are common to most or all types of violence and which are specific to particular forms of violence.

Increase the Developmental Focus of Research

As described in Chap. 4, there are developmental antecedents to all forms of inter-personal violence, and exposure to abuse, maltreatment, and other forms of trauma increases vulnerability to later victimization as well as perpetration of violence. Broad models encompassing many forms of violence and models that are narrower in scope will need to consider the temporal relations among them. For example, work on the sequelae of childhood experiences of maltreatment and family violence could explicitly address the processes by which they contribute to the most common forms of aggression in middle childhood and adolescence (e.g., bullying, dating violence, and sexual harassment). More precise knowledge about the developmental trajecto-ries of different types of violence and how they wax and wane in tandem with one another also would inform models of co-occurrence. For example, Moffitt's concepts of adolescence-limited delinquency and life-course-persistent delinquency (1993), which already focus on developmental patterns more than most models of violence, could be expanded to look at how delinquent behavior intersects with victimization experiences. This framework also could be used to distinguish between peer, fam-ily, and community targets of perpetration, and the antecedents of different types of perpetration, such as the commission of sexual assaults versus physical assaults. A developmental approach also would focus more attention on peak age periods for certain types of violence involvement and take greater account of chronicity.

Although we have emphasized the connections among different forms of vio-lence in this book, it is just as important to understand discontinuity as continu-ity. How do some children who have grown up in abusive and violent homes avoid becoming perpetrators or victims in other relationships? As powerful as experiences with violence are, especially early in life, there are other powerful forces that can counteract their adverse effects. Unfortunately, we know relatively little about them. Research on resilience has identified several classes of constructs associated with good outcomes in children exposed to adversity (Masten and Coatsworth 1998), but how they function is not well understood. A developmental focus in research on violence can help identify key windows for intervention and even explore whether the malleability of some risk factors also changes over the course of the lifespan.

Attend More to the Linkages Between Victimization and Perpetration

There are some well-known models of the links between victimization and perpetra-tion, such as the intergenerational transmission of violence (Widom and White 1997) and the concept of bully victims (Salmivalli and Nieminen 2002). More needs to be done, however, to recognize that perpetrator-victims are one of the most common types of involvement in violence, if not the most common type. As has been noted elsewhere (Hamby and Gray-Little 2007; Loseke 1992), the field is still strongly influenced by societal stereotypes about monstrous perpetrators and virtuous victims. These over simplified, two-dimensional depictions may satisfy desires for a just world, but they do not accurately depict the lives of many people and how they become caught up in violence. Aggression and even violence are often used to try to meet needs that are not, in and of themselves, maladaptive, problematic, or wrong. Most aggressive youths and adults have the same desires to feel included, respected, powerful, and in at least partial control of their environment. As Chap. 4 showed, in many cases aggression arises out of a history of maltreatment and trauma, and the processes that lead to aggressive behavior (e.g., hypersensitivity to signs of anger) may have played a protective or adaptive role in one context or at one time.

Relatedly, although there are instances in which 100 % of the variance in victimization is due to transitory situational factors (namely, the behavior of the perpetrator in the situation), there is sufficient evidence to show that there are chronic factors, some environmental and some individual, that make some people vulnerable to being victimized repeatedly. Recognizing this empirical fact is not victim blaming. In fact, we argue that ignoring these factors is irresponsible, because it prevents identification of strategies that could prevent future victimization. Perpetrating victims and victimized perpetrators also suffer with each and every additional involvement in violence, as much as if not more than those with less extensive involvement in violence. Dyadic models that incorporate the characteristics and behavior of both parties in an aggressive interaction hold considerable promise for understanding the interpersonal nature of relationship violence (e.g., Capaldi and Kim 2007; Card 2011). A more nuanced, contextualized depiction of perpetrator-victims might not only enhance our understanding of violence but also help us make better intervention decisions in situations where a comprehensive, person-centered assessment indicates that clear lines between perpetrator and victim may be hard to draw.

Design Methods to Advance the Science of Co-occurrence

The interconnections among types of violence also have significant implications for designing studies that investigate violence in one or more contexts. Decisions about who is studied, what is measured, and how data are analyzed and interpreted will shape the potential for future research to offer insight into how and why different types of violence co-occur.

Sampling

The decision about who to study is important for all studies, and it has particularly critical implications for research on co-occurrence. Participants recruited using different strategies are likely to differ in their rates and types of co-occurrence and severity of the violence that they have experienced. These differences, in turn, thus may lead to different conclusions about the causes and consequences of violence. Both the degree of co-occurrence and the severity of particular forms of violence are higher in at-risk samples than community samples (Cyr et al., in press). For example, children and adolescents recruited through Child Protective Services or clinical settings are likely to have more extensive histories of co-occurrence as well as severe forms of at least one form of maltreatment or exposure to violence than unselected community samples. Further, severity and degree of co-occurrence may be related, such that victims of prolonged and severe abuse are more likely to have experienced other forms of maltreatment and violence. Extent of co-occurrence also may be related to other factors such as poverty and broader family dysfunction. The impact of systematic differences in rates and severity are well known in research on intimate partner violence, where research utilizing samples recruited through agencies serving battered women often has led to different conclusions about the nature and extent of violence than samples drawn from the community. However, we will not know how variations in patterns of co-occurrence influence development until they are measured and tested. Studies that assess the same constructs with similar methods in samples recruited from different populations could provide valuable insight into these questions.

A related issue is that selecting a sample based on one type of violence does not always mean that this form of violence is the most salient or significant one they have experienced. Researchers interested in physical abuse may recruit participants through CPS, find that physical abuse is associated with a range of adverse effects, and conclude that physical abuse is the cause. Another researcher interested in sexual abuse may study the same sample, focus on documenting sexual abuse, and conclude that sexual abuse is the cause of adverse outcomes. Although different forms of violence may well have unique effects, it is possible that the most adverse type of violence is the one that has been most severe or prolonged. Alternatively, it may be that the number or duration of experiences rather than any particular type best explains psychological adjustment, as has been found in NatSCEV (Turner et al. 2010). It is also possible that the relative or additive impacts might vary depending on the particular outcome under study. These situations underscore the importance of thoroughly assessing participants' experiences with violence other than the one that is the focus of the study. We are not suggesting that all forms of violence have the same antecedents and consequences, but we will not know which predictors and outcomes are specific to particular forms unless we carefully measure and examine multiple types. Depending on the question being investigated, different sampling strategies will be more or less appropriate for drawing valid conclusions from the data.

Design Issues

An approach that may appear to lead to valid conclusions about the unique effects of a particular form of violence involves isolating that form by design. A group of potential participants could be screened, and only participants who have experienced the type of violence that is the focus of the study and only that type could be included. An example would be a study that identifies victims of child sexual abuse who had not also been exposed to intimate partner violence, neglect, bullying, or other violence, and then compares them to children who have not been sexually abused. Although this comparison may seem to provide a test of the specific effects of child abuse, it does not, at least not if the sequelae of sexual abuse are shared by other forms of violence. More accurate conclusions could be drawn if a third comparison group were added: children without a history of child abuse who have experienced other forms of violence. Another limitation of this approach to isolating the effects of a particular type of violence is that the results will generalize only to those who have experienced a particular form of abuse without exposure to other types of violence, which, as we described in Chap. 2, does not represent the majority of victims.

An alternative to screening participants based on their exposure or nonexposure to particular types of violence is to measure a variety of forms of violence and then examine their interrelations and associations with other constructs of interest. This approach has the advantage of assessing covariation among the forms as they occur naturally, and thus maximizes generalizability. The potential disadvantage is in interpreting the effects of a particular form of violence when it is intercorrelated with other forms; however, attempting to isolate the effects of a construct when it is not naturally isolated will not enhance our understanding of the phenomenon. Although for some purposes it may be useful to attempt to isolate effects, if reality is complex, ultimately our models of violence must reflect and attend to that complexity.

Measurement

It is not feasible for every study to obtain a detailed assessment of every type of interpersonal violence participants may have experienced, but there are workable strategies that would expand the focus of research. One approach would be to use brief screening measures for multiple types of violence, such as the Juvenile Victimization Questionnaire (Finkelhor et al. 2005), the Adverse Childhood Experiences questionnaire (Felitti et al. 1998), or the National Intimate and Sexual Violence Survey (Black et al. 2011). Even knowing whether a particular form occurred, or better yet, its frequency, would be useful. Alternatively, studies could focus on a narrower set of forms (those that are closely linked theoretically or empirically) and assess those forms more thoroughly.

Another measurement implication is the need to develop more precise measures of violence. Many measures of violence use fairly general terms such as "abuse" in the items of the survey that could refer to many different types of violent or aggressive behaviors. Some focus on specific types of perpetrators, whereas others do not specifically indicate any type of victim-offender relationship. Although progress has been made in the widespread adoption of more behaviorally specific items, virtually all survey measures of violence are influenced by respondents' self-perceptions of themselves as victim or perpetrator and willingness to disclose. This creates problems for studies that seek to assess both perpetration and victimization, because perpetration is under-reported in comparison to victimization. It can also be challenging to compare forms that are more stigmatized to those that are less stigmatized. We need to know much more about the consequences of these different measurement decisions, especially for the comparable assessment of acts that range from bullying to caregiver-perpetrated sexual assault.

The field of violence has barely delved into standard measures of assessment quality, such as sensitivity and specificity. The few exceptions in this regard, such as the Child Abuse Potential Inventory (Milner and Crouch, 2012), provide one model for approaching this issue. Although a true gold standard may be hard to obtain due to the private nature of most violence, much more use of multi-method approaches are needed in general and will be even more important for exploring the interrelationships among different forms of violence. These multi-method approaches could include the use of multiple informants, more use of electronic diary-based or other microlongitudinal approaches and greater use of official or archival records. The development of questionnaires that more specifically assess different types of violence, in ways that map onto official and institutional uses in law enforcement, child protection, schools, and elsewhere, is also much needed. As discussed in Chap. 2, we should strive for a multi-method approach to the study of violence. Ideally, we will consistently identify rates and risk factors across forms of violence, but at a minimum we need a clear understanding about the consequences of different methodological choices.

Improving Distinctions Between Limited and Severe Violence

An increased understanding of co-occurrence would be enhanced by a better understanding of limited versus extensive or severe involvement in violence. Although the study of co-occurrence can proceed with an all-or-none approach to classification, this approach has limitations. Some exposure to violence as perpetrator, victim, or both is a nearly universal experience, especially when verbal aggression, social exclusion, or other noncontact assaults are included, but the concept of co-occurrence is less useful if it is broadened to a point where it includes the entire population.

The most likely means of accomplishing this is to build some thresholds into measurement. This can be done along at least two dimensions, severity, and frequency. A severity threshold can exclude the most trivial events, and a frequency threshold can exclude the rarest ones. Different thresholds will be needed for different types of violence. A frequency threshold, for example, would obviously be inappropriate for rape, but it may be appropriate for verbal aggression. Some offenses, such as neglect, have frequency built into the very concept—a single missed meal or late vaccination does not make one a neglectful parent as the concept is usually applied. Thresholds can also be used to avoid labeling people for minor and infrequent acts, or for diluting the meaning of important constructs. For example, some research on intimate partner violence uses terms like "batterer" for a group that is primarily composed of individuals who have slapped or pushed their partner one or two times. This is not what the general public means when they say "batterer," and we should be cautious about greatly broadening the definition of emotionally laden, stigmatizing terms (Hamby and Gray-Little 2000). In sum, the study of co-occurrence will require much more careful operationalization of constructs, and much more attention to how they map onto important institutional and societal uses of violence terms.

Data Analysis

The recommendation to expand the focus of studies of violence to encompass multiple types of violence creates analytic challenges. It entails increasing the number of predictor or response variables being studied, some of which may be nested within different levels of analysis (e.g., children within families within neighborhoods), and placing greater emphasis on following participants over time. These implications for design and methodology in turn require larger samples and more complex data analytic strategies. For example, when violence is being examined as a predictor, it will be important to consider both the additive and interactive effects of the forms being studied, and testing interactions sensitively requires considerable power as well as sufficient range and variability on the variables included in the interaction term (McClelland and Judd 1993). One common approach to handling multiple predictors is to try to isolate the effects of one variable by statistically controlling interrelated variables, but this approach has both conceptual and statistical problems (Cook and Campbell 1979; Steinberg and Fletcher 1998). Furthermore, if the goal is to understand how multiple factors are interrelated, then "controlling" the ones that are of less interest in a given study in order to focus on those of greater interest is counterproductive. Rather than attempting to control certain variables, we recommend an "assess and analyze" approach; that is, measure the constructs that might be important and empirically test which have unique or joint effects.

A number of sophisticated approaches to analyzing such complex data have been developed. Multilevel modeling (MLM) includes a family of statistical models (e.g., hierarchical linear models, covariance structure analyses, and growth curve analysis) that are designed for analyzing variables that are nested within multiple levels (e.g., children within families, families within communities), collected over time, or both (Luke 2004; Raudenbush and Bryk 2002). Variables that are clustered or nested hierarchically tend to be correlated and consequently create difficulties for interpreting the results of statistical methods that assume independence (specifically, they increase the likelihood of Type 1 errors, or incorrectly concluding that significant effects exist when they do not). For example, Javdani et al. (2011) recently examined how the presence of coordinating councils in the community impact important indicators of system change; specifically, judicial referrals to domestic violence shelters and issuance of protective orders. They examined how the rates of referrals and protective orders varied across 21 judicial circuits in the US over the course of 15 years with and without coordinating councils. In this case, referrals and protective orders are clustered within judicial circuits, and likely are correlated with other characteristics of those circuits. Using MLM, Javdani et al. (2011) found that there was a general trend for protection orders to increase over time, but that this trend occurred only in geographic regions that had established coordinating councils; further, the amount of time that the council had been in existence was related to the rate of protective orders issued in that circuit. In contrast, referrals to domestic violence agencies varied across circuits but did not change over time.

The variable-centered statistical approaches most often used in violence (and most other) research also may inadvertently contribute to compartmentalization in the study of interpersonal violence. By describing the frequency and covariation of different forms of violent behavior *across* a sample, variable-centered analyses do not indicate which forms co-occur *within* the individuals studied. Consequently, they do not take into consideration the fact a particular form of violence or a particular process is embedded within a broader constellation of factors that may influence how that form (or forms) of violence relates to child functioning. For example, the experience of being bullied might have a different effect for children who also have experienced maltreatment or witnessed intimate partner violence, and beliefs about the justifiability of dating violence may have a different impact in individuals who also have poor emotion regulation and narcissistic personality traits than individuals without those qualities.

A second approach to analyzing complex, clustered data is represented by person-centered analytical approaches. These approaches can be used to assess the configuration of particular characteristics within individuals, and are best suited for capturing qualitative, nonlinear differences between individuals; consequently, they offer an alternative perspective to variable-based approaches. Cluster and latent class analyses have proven useful in describing homogeneous subgroups in research on some forms of interpersonal violence. For example, research on bullying has documented reliable differences in children who bully, those who are victimized, and those who are both bullies and victims (e.g., Espelage and Holt 2007). Methods have also been developed that combine statistical approaches, such as latent class growth analysis, which uses advanced modeling techniques to track how different subgroups of perpetrators or victims change over time (e.g., Swartout et al. 2011).

Although these approaches offer a more holistic approach to studying violence, any approach has its limitations. For example, research on intimate partner violence has led to a number of person-centered classification schemes (e.g., common couple violence vs. intimate terrorism), but the validity of the resulting subtypes has been questioned, and the evidence that they capture stable groups of people who differ reliably on particular dimensions is mixed (e.g., Capaldi and Kim 2007). Any given solution is a product of the specific variables included in the analysis and can change significantly with the addition or deletion of particular measures. It is important that the choice of variables is conceptually guided, and that the classification scheme is validated by demonstrating that resulting groups are distinguished by theoretically meaningful criteria. Further, the groups that emerge from these analyses also must be cross-validated in new samples to increase confidence in their reliability and validity, and if they are assumed to be stable over time, evaluated longitudinally. The broader solution, as in most areas of research, is to utilize a variety of methodological and data analytic approaches across studies. Both variable- and person-oriented methods have something to offer the study of interpersonal violence; by providing different perspectives on the same phenomena, they will enrich our understanding of the connections among different forms of violence.

Conclusion

There are numerous feasible and relatively straightforward approaches that could vastly improve our understanding of the co-occurrence of violence. Conceptual models that focus explicitly on co-occurrence are needed to guide empirical research; although these models may vary in their scope, they will function to identify common factors across types of violence as well as factors specific to particular forms, describe their developmental trajectories, and deepen understanding of the links between perpetration and victimization. Even minor modifications to existing approaches, steps as simple as adding a questionnaire that screens for multiple types of violence, can lead to a more valid and comprehensive knowledge base and improve research on interpersonal violence. In this chapter, we have focused primarily on the conceptual and technological needs for advancing our basic understanding of co-occurrence. In the next chapter, we take up the issue of using an appreciation of co-occurrence as a means of advancing prevention, clinical assessment, and intervention against multiple forms of violence.

References

Anderson, C. A., & Bushman, B. J. (2002). Human aggression. *Annual Review of Psychology, 53*, 27–51.

Black, M., Basile, K., Breiding, M., Smith, S., Walters, M., Merrick, M., et al. (2011). *The national intimate and sexual violence survey: 2010 summary report.* Atlanta: Centers for Disease Control and Prevention.

Capaldi, D., & Kim, H. (2007). Typological approaches to violence in couples: A critique and alternative conceptual approach. *Clinical Psychology Review, 27*, 253–265.

Card, N. (2011). Toward a relationship perspective on aggression among schoolchildren: Integrating social cognitive and interdependence theories. *Psychology of Violence, 1*(3), 188–201.

Ciardha, C., & Gannon, T. (2011). The cognitive distortions of child molesters are in need of treatment. *Journal of Sexual Aggression, 17*(2), 130–141.

Cook, T. D., & Campbell, D. T. (1979). *Quasi-experimentation: Design and analysis issues for field settings*. Boston: Houghton-Mifflin.

Espelage, D., & Holt, M. (2007). Dating violence and sexual harassment across the bully-victim continuum among middle and high school students. *Journal of Youth and Adolescence, 36,* 799–811.

Felitti, V. J., Anda, R. F., Nordenberg, D., Williamson, D. F., Spitz, A. M., Edwards, V., et al. (1998). Relationship of childhood abuse and household dysfunction to many of the leading causes of death in adults. *American Journal of Preventive Medicine, 14*(4), 245–258.

Finkel, E. (2008). Intimate partner violence perpetration: Insights from the science of self-regulation. In J. Forgas & J. Fitness (Eds.), *Social relationships: Cognitive, affective, and motivational processes*. New York: Psychology Press.

Finkel, E., DeWall, C. N., Slotter, E. B., Oaten, M., & Foshee, V. A. (2009). Self-regulatory failure and intimate partner violence perpetration. *Journal of Personality and Social Psychology, 97*(3), 483–499. doi:Doi10.1037/A0015433.

Finkelhor, D., Hamby, S., Ormrod, R., & Turner, H. (2005). The juvenile victimization questionnaire: Reliability, validity, and national norms. *Child Abuse and Neglect, 29,* 383–412.

Gannon, T., Ward, T., Beech, A., & Fisher, D. (2007). *Aggressive offenders' cognition: Theory, research and practice*. New York: Wiley.

Gilbert, F., & Daffern, M. (2010). Integrating contemporary aggression theory with violent offender treatment: How thoroughly do interventions target violent behavior? *Aggression and Violent Behavior, 15,* 167–180.

Grych, J. H., & Kinsfogel, K. (2010). Exploring the role of attachment style in the relation between family aggression and abuse in adolescent dating relationships. *Journal of Aggression, Maltreatment, and Trauma, 19,* 624–664.

Hamby, S., & Gray-Little, B. (2000). Labeling partner violence: When do victims differentiate among acts? *Violence and Victims, 15*(2), 173–186.

Hamby, S., & Gray-Little, B. (2007). Can battered women cope? A critical analysis of research on women's responses to violence. In K. Kendall-Tackett & S. Giacomoni (Eds.), *Intimate partner violence*. Kingston: Civic Research Institute.

Hamby, S., Finkelhor, D., Turner, H., & Ormrod, R. (2010). The overlap of witnessing partner violence with child maltreatment and other victimizations in a nationally representative survey of youth. *Child Abuse and Neglect, 34,* 734–741.

Holtzworth-Munroe, A., & Stuart, G. L. (1994). Typologies of male batterers: Three subtypes and the differences among them. Psychological Bulletin, *116,* 476–497.

Javdani, S., Allen, N. E., Todd, N. R., & Anderson, C. J. (2011). Examining systems change in the response to domestic violence: Innovative applications of multilevel modeling. *Violence Against Women, 17*(3), 359–375. doi:10.1177/1077801211398621.

Jouriles, E., Grych, J. H., McDonald, R., Rosenfield, D., & Dodson, M. C. (2011). Automatic cognitions and teen dating violence. *Psychology of Violence, 1*(4), 302–314. doi:10.1037/a0025157.

Loseke, D. R. (1992). *The battered woman and shelters: The social construction of wife abuse*. Albany: State University of New York Press.

Luke, D. A. (2004). *Multilevel modeling*. Thousand Oaks: Sage.

Masten, A., & Coatsworth, J. (1998). The development of competence in favorable and unfavorable environments: Lessons from research on successful children. *American Psychologist, 53,* 205–220.

McClelland, G., & Judd, C. (1993). Statistical difficulties of detecting interactions and moderator effects. *Psychological Bulletin, 114,* 376–389.

Milner, J. S., & Crouch, J. L. (2012). Psychometric characteristics of translated versions of the Child Abuse Potential Inventory. *Psychology of Violence, 2*(3), 239–259. doi: 10.1037/a0026957

Raudenbush, S., & Bryk, A. (2002). *Hierarchical linear models: Applications and data analysis methods*. Thousand Oaks: Sage.

Repetti, R., Robles, T., & Reynolds, B. (2011). Allostatic processes in the family. *Development and Psychopathology, 23,* 921–938.

Rothman, E., Johnson, R., Azrael, D., Hall, D., & Weinberg, J. (2010). Perpetration of physical assault among dating partners, peers, and siblings among a locally representative sample of high school students in Boston, Massachusetts. *Archives of Pediatric and Adolescent Medicine, 164*(12), 1118–1124.

Salmivalli, C., & Nieminen, E. (2002). Proactive and reactive aggression among school bullies, victims, and bully-victims. *Aggressive Behavior, 28*(1), 30–44.

Steinberg, L., & Fletcher, A. (1998). Data analytic strategies on research on ethnic minority youth. In V. McLoyd & L. Steinberg (Eds.), *Studying minority adolesents mahwah*. NJ: Erlbaum.

Swartout, K. M., Swartout, A. G., & White, J. W. (2011). A person-centered, longitudinal approach to sexual victimization. *Psychology of Violence, 1*(1), 29–40. doi:10.1037/a0022069.

Turner, H., Finkelhor, D., & Ormrod, R. (2010). Poly-victimization in a national sample of children and youth. *American Journal of Preventive Medicine, 38*(3), 323–330.

Widom, C., & White, H. R. (1997). Problem behaviours in abused and neglected children grown up: Prevalence and co-occurrence of substance abuse, crime and violence. *Criminal Behavior and Mental Health, 7*, 287–310.

Chapter 6
Implications for Prevention and Intervention: A More Person-Centered Approach

One of the most important functions of any theoretical framework is to guide practice in the field. The accumulated data on co-occurrence provide strong evidence that prevention and intervention of all types of violence should be organized around the full context of individuals' experiences, not narrowly defined subtypes of abuse or violence. The research discussed in previous chapters provides new urgency to calls to better integrate victim services. Additionally, services aimed at perpetrators or would-be perpetrators of particular violence types could be more effective, if they address the fact that many perpetrators offend in multiple contexts and often have victimization histories. In this chapter, we discuss how recognizing the interrelations among different forms of violence can guide prevention, assessment, and intervention.

Prevention

How Compartmentalization Affects Prevention

Traditionally, prevention is the area that has had perhaps the most siloed approach. There are programs for bullying prevention, dating violence prevention, and sexual assault prevention. There are programs to discourage gang involvement and reduce youth homicide. There are programs that attempt to prevent child abuse against young children that are distinct from efforts to prevent intimate partner violence in recently married couples. Programs teach younger children to avoid potential sexual predators, but not other dangerous adults or youth. When forms of violence catch the public's attention, more specific programs are developed. For example, there are now cyber bullying interventions that are distinct from other bullying prevention efforts. Further, these programs typically are offered in isolation from programs on key modifiable risk factors for violence, such as substance abuse and teen pregnancy.

S. Hamby and J. Grych, *The Web of Violence*, SpringerBriefs in Sociology,
DOI: 10.1007/978-94-007-5596-3_6, © The Author(s) 2013

Despite the nominal intention to address different problems areas, however, there is considerable overlap across these programs in both their content and methods. Effective prevention programs share certain characteristics regardless of their intended target (Nation et al. 2003). They emphasize building positive, respectful relationships rather than simply trying to reduce undesirable behaviors, teach life skills such as problem solving, conflict resolution, and communication, and often include guidance on how to recognize and avoid risky situations and utilize effective "refusal skills". Many of them attempt to dispel attitudes or myths that promote violence, and although some of these are specific to certain kinds of violence, the counter messages are often similar and generally espouse nonviolent, egalitarian values. Most promote help-seeking if violence is encountered. The curricular approaches also are similar, with most classroom curricula organized around role-plays, analysis of scenarios presented in videos and vignettes, and use of self-assessment questionnaires of values and attitudes. Newer "social marketing" programs primarily use media to raise awareness, create positive shifts in community norms, and promote desired behaviors such as bystander interventions and help-seeking (Potter 2012). The majority target young people in a fairly narrow developmental period from middle school to young adulthood.

The overlapping content of many prevention programs implicitly acknowledges that different types of violence have similar etiologies, as we have shown in Chap. 3. Explicitly recognizing this similarity and systematically incorporating common factors into comprehensive prevention programs can increase the efficiency and impact of prevention efforts.

Improving Prevention Through Greater Emphasis on Co-occurrence

The advantages of addressing multiple components and domains have been consistently demonstrated in a small subset of prevention programs that are aimed at a variety of youth problems (Nation et al. 2003). There are promising efforts to develop more comprehensive approaches that could serve as models for improving prevention. For example, although the Fourth R (Wolfe et al. 2009) emphasizes dating violence prevention as its primary goal, it addresses dating violence in the context of peer violence, substance use, and the onset of sexual activity. Some programs address both dating and sexual violence, including many bystander prevention programs (Banyard 2011) and "Shifting Boundaries," which has both classroom and school-wide program elements (Taylor et al. 2011). "Youth violence prevention" programs (Thornton et al. 2002) try to reduce involvement in many violence forms, usually by trying to reduce the perpetration of delinquency and peer violence.

Still, these efforts to integrate across violence types are relatively new, and they tend to focus on what have historically been viewed as related problems, such as gang involvement and general delinquency, or dating and sexual violence. Perhaps the best evidence that prevention programs can affect diverse forms of violent behavior comes from youth violence programs that target multiple types of delinquency (Thornton et al. 2002). There is less evidence for the effects of programs addressing dating or sexual violence, especially for changes in perpetration or victimization versus attitudes or knowledge. For example, in its first published evaluation, the Fourth R reduced dating violence perpetration for boys but had no effect on peer violence, substance use, or condom use (Wolfe et al. 2009). Still, the fact that it showed any impact on aggression at all makes it one of the best-supported dating violence prevention programs. Safe Dates has reduced both physical and sexual aggression, but thus far has only has examined aggression in dating relationships (Foshee et al. 2000). Shifting Boundaries' school-wide interventions (more security at violence "hotspots" and posters to raise awareness, for example) focused on dating violence, but more consistently reduced peer sexual victimization (Taylor et al. 2011).

Next Steps: Advancing Prevention Through Explicit Emphasis on Co-occurrence

1. *Develop a prevention framework that programatically addresses common factors.* The value of prevention now is widely recognized, and many youths in the US participate in as many as three or four programs in school settings. In most ways, this is a good thing. However, the proliferation of prevention programs has at least one potentially unintended effect. As we described earlier, programs created to address a variety of different problems present similar content in similar ways. Consequently, there may be duplication across programs that leads students to "tune out" after a while. Indeed, this high level of repetition may be one reason why only 17 % of a college student sample found the material in prevention curricula to be helpful, and 70 % said they already knew the information that was covered (Chandrasekaran and Hamby 2010). Research showing that a common set of risk factors is associated with diverse types of interpersonal violence supports the value of focusing on these factors in programs targeting different kinds of problem, but it is possible to do so in a coordinated, planful way that adapts the message to the developmental phase and social ecology relevant at different ages (Kazdin and Blase 2011). Prevention programs could parallel the way that math is taught in many schools: basic mathematical concepts are introduced early in elementary school, and are revisited, expanded, and tailored to different topics as children learn algebra, geometry and trigonometry in middle and high school.

What would a programatic, school-based approach to preventing interpersonal violence look like? It would address the cognitive, emotional, behavioral, and even physiologic processes described in Chap. 3 in developmentally appropriate ways, adapting them to different relationship contexts as they become salient. More concretely, teaching communication and conflict resolution skills, fostering empathy, and promoting emotional and behavioral self-regulation are likely to reduce many forms of perpetration, and we believe that a core curriculum could be developed that includes these skills and is supported by strategies used in social marketing campaigns to promote nonviolent community norms. Prevention programing could begin in elementary school by focusing first on treating peers with respect and kindness. Although some children may begin school with positive attitudes about aggression, establishing a school culture that emphasizes social inclusion and peaceful solutions to conflict would send a strong and consistent counter-message. This foundation would set the stage for addressing issues pertinent to bullying, harassment, and relational aggression. Many youths engage in bullying and sexual harassment to increase their social status or power, but this strategy only works if the behavior actually is rewarded by peers. Creating a culture that does not tolerate aggression could remove this source of reinforcement, and incorporating principles from bystander interventions programs would further strengthen this effect. Teaching anger regulation strategies and assertiveness also could strengthen forces that inhibit aggressive impulses and make potential victims harder targets. Later, when romantic relationships become salient, relationship skills could be expanded to include attention to new kinds of intimacy and the feelings that they can engender (e.g., jealousy, resentment) and assertive resistance strategies.

Although this program emphasizes factors common to most forms of violence, it also could include unique risk factors and dynamics that are associated with specific forms of violence. These could be addressed in special topics modules that build on the core curriculum but do not duplicate it. For example, modules for dating violence and sexual assault might include navigating sexual consent and negotiating birth control use. Dealing with gang-involved peers or coping with school social hierarchies might also warrant specialized modules. See Fig. 6.1 for one possible model of how these common and specific factors might be integrated into one broader, more coordinated program.

2. *Incorporate knowledge on intersecting developmental trajectories.* Although prevention programs tend to be most effective when they target topics that are salient to youths but have not yet developed into notable problems, the building blocks for interpersonal violence often are in place well before experiences like dating are on their radar. As Chap. 4 showed, the roots of most violence are found in early relationships or environments in which children's needs are ignored or dismissed, and are intensified when they experience demeaning or abusive behavior at the hands of parents and peers. Consequently, it is difficult to imagine how early universal prevention programs would need to start to include groups of children with no victimization history. Similarly, developmental research shows that aggressive behavior typically peaks during the toddler years and then steadily decreases (Coté et al. 2006), and so prevention is not something that can be offered before children have ever engaged in aggression. One could argue that effective prevention of bullying, dating violence, and other aggression begins when parents provide caring and consistent care to their infants and toddlers, and is further strengthened when schools and other societal institutions join parents in promoting respect and compassion in early peer relationships. Virtually all children aggress against peers at some point in time, and so the real task of "prevention" is ensuring that control

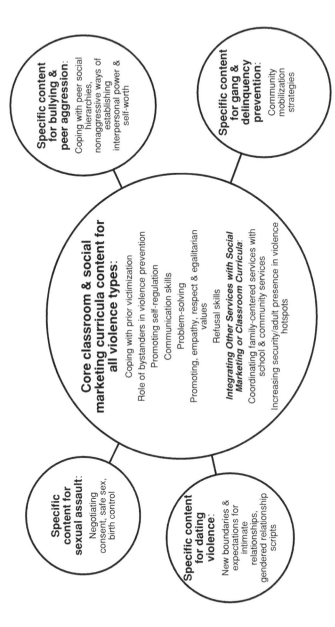

Note This model focuses on violence prevention among youth. Similar models could be applied to other key populations, such as new parents or newly married couples. Given the lack of empirical data on effective curricular elements (see section on *Identifying the "active ingredients" of effective programs*), this model is purely hypothetical

Fig. 6.1 Coordinated Violence Prevention Model: Hypothetical Common and Specific Elements

over aggressive impulses increases as rapidly as possible and that the normal limits to coping with frustration and anger which characterize most toddlers do not develop into serious and persistent aggressive behaviors.

Recent epidemiologic research shows that different victimization types have different developmental trajectories. Bullying, for example, peaks in middle school and declines through later adolescence. Sexual victimization, on the other hand, rises steadily across the span of childhood, especially for girls (Finkelhor et al. 2009). For girls, risk of sexual assault remains high through young adulthood, whereas boys may be most vulnerable to rape under the age of 12 (Tjaden and Thoennes 2006). Exposure to community violence rises steadily and increases markedly when youth enter adolescence (Finkelhor et al. 2009). These findings underscore the importance of timing prevention offerings and paying more attention to early experiences, especially experiences of victimization or neglect.

Early home visitation is another developmentally attuned violence prevention strategy. Support for parents and toddlers may be the single most important means of preventing multiple forms of violence. Helping parents to recognize and respond to their children's needs and to use effective discipline strategies provides a foundation for healthy and safe interpersonal relationships. Studies of programs such as the Nurse Family Partnership show early home visitation can substantially decrease child maltreatment (Olds 2006). In the US, the recently signed Affordable Care Act will significantly expand early home visitation and offer a vehicle for delivering prevention programing at a crucial developmental time period.

3. *Address history of violence exposure in prevention programs.* The developmental nature of interpersonal violence indicates that prevention effects are likely to be diluted if they do not address the sequelae of early family and other childhood experiences. Early childhood victimization can lead to neurophysiologic changes that create conditions of hyper- or hypoarousal in stressful interpersonal situations (De Bellis 2001; Repetti et al. 2011). This suggests that prevention programs need to teach youth how to respond in highly stressful situations when they may be experiencing overarousal or underarousal (Noll and Grych 2011). Some evidence suggests that prevention programs are less effective for the most violent subgroup of youth. For example, Foshee and colleagues (2005) found that youths who reported engaging in high levels of dating aggression prior to participating in the Safe Dates program did not show any changes in perpetration of severe violence; only those with no or low levels of prior dating aggression reported lower rates of physical and sexual violence after participating in the program.

We propose that common therapeutic interventions, such as cognitive restructuring, anger management, grounding, and mindfulness meditation, could be adapted for universal prevention programs. For some, classroom-based prevention alone may not be sufficient to alter their behavior. More intensive interventions addressing the cognitive, emotional, and physiologic processes believed to lead to violence will be needed, which may involve both individual and family services. Expect Respect does this by adding a more therapeutic adjunct, in the form of a group for victimized youth (Ball et al. 2009). School-based prevention could also be enhanced by adding components that address parenting and family issues. For example, Dishion and Stormshak's (2007) EcoFIT model is a multilevel middle school program that establishes a family resource center at the school. In addition to conducting peer groups in the school, parents are offered the "Family Check-up", which involves assessment of their children and families' strengths and needs and feedback utilizing motivational interviewing techniques. Interested parents can receive phone "check-ins" or participate in individual or group-based family management training at the school. Although EcoFIT does not focus on violence, it provides an empirically supported model for offering family-centered services within the context of school programing (Dishion and Stormshak 2007; Stormshak and Dishion 2009). Notably, in contrast to Safe Dates' findings, the effects of EcoFIT have been strongest on youths with the most severe adjustment problems (Connell et al. 2007).

Challenges in Making Prevention More Informed by Co-occurrence

Identifying the "active ingredients" of effective programs. To achieve a large goal, such as reducing violence, it is important to break the task down into component steps and evaluate each step. When the US wanted to send an astronaut to the moon, NASA first tested a variety of different rocket boosters, developed spacecraft to withstand the atmosphere, tested new navigational systems with shorter missions such as orbiting the Earth, explored the effects of weightlessness on the human body, and developed and tested space suits that would protect astronauts from the vacuum of space (to name just a few required tasks). They did not put the astronauts into their best guesses about each of these components, light up a rocket and hope for the best. Even in the case of catastrophic failures such as the Challenger accident, it was readily understood that the task of the subsequent investigation was to identify which component failed, not to decide whether the space program as a whole did or did not "work".

Unfortunately, prevention programs most often have been developed, evaluated, disseminated, and sold as fully formed entities. Even in cases where a particular program has demonstrated behavioral effects on violence, the research does not indicate which elements produce the change. Some curricular elements could be having no effect, or worse, negative (aka "backlash") effects that are outweighed by effective elements (as found, for example, in Jaffe et al. 1992; Taylor et al. 2011). This becomes especially problematic because schools that adopt these programs often make changes to suit their local circumstances; they might have to condense the program into fewer hours, or choose between implementing the social marketing piece or the classroom curricula. Unfortunately, because there is virtually no research on which components are effective, there is no empirical basis for deciding which components to keep and which to drop if a whole program cannot be implemented.

This problem is particularly pertinent for developing an integrated approach to prevention that addresses multiple types of violence. At this point, we can only speculate about which elements should be retained in a coordinated strategy. This is true at the broadest levels, such as the relative merits of classroom curricula versus social marketing campaigns, and at more specific levels, such as which elements of classroom curricula are most essential or have the broadest impact. For example, the near universal inclusion of some form of conflict resolution and negotiation skills (Thornton et al. 2002; Wolfe et al. 2009) suggests that these skills are widely perceived to be a key element of healthy relationships, but we do not know if teaching these skills directly reduces violence or if the benefits of programs that include them are due to something else, such as raising awareness or changing social norms. Taylor et al. (2011) found that a program comprising school-wide interventions (such as increasing faculty presence at violence "hotspots" and a poster campaign to raise awareness and help-seeking) significantly decreased some types of violence, while a classroom-based curriculum did not. One cannot tell, however, which school-wide intervention led to the effect (was security more important than the public awareness campaign?). Even more notably, while the school-wide program appeared to reduce some types of violence, others actually increased. Lack of a curricular analysis makes it impossible to tell not only which elements accounted for the change but whether there might be some combination of elements that could avoid an iatrogenic effect.

The time afforded to these programs during the school day is too valuable to be spent doing things that are not helpful or may even have negative effects. Simply going with adults' perceptions of helpful content is not sufficient. These same points also apply to other programs such as early home visitation, which are often combined with parenting groups, enhanced early childhood education through Head Start, or other mechanisms. We need carefully designed studies that evaluate each curricular component and, eventually, begin to identify the most powerful combination of effective components.

The dose issue. Related to the problem of not knowing which program elements have the greatest impact is the problem of not knowing how much of these elements to provide. Although it is widely acknowledged that one-time efforts are unlikely to have a lasting impact (e.g., Anderson and Whiston 2005), there is room to be much more precise than "more than one session." For example, when Safe Dates (Foshee et al. 1996) was adapted for the Canadian school curriculum (Wolfe et al. 2009), content related to substance abuse and contraception was added and the number of sessions was raised from 9 to 21. Both programs showed effects and are among the best validated dating violence prevention programs. But there is little evidence that 21 sessions was markedly better than 9. Indeed, the 9-session program showed significant improvements for both boys and girls, and the 21-session version only for boys. This should not be taken as evidence that 9 is a magic number—we do not know how it compares to 10 or 8 or 40. The effective dose also may be age related; it is possible that the effective number of hours for a particular component differs for youths of different ages. Classroom curricula are expensive, labor-intensive programs, and all things being equal, it is better to implement effective short programs in more schools and more classrooms than longer programs in fewer schools.

The scalability issue. The widespread involvement in multiple forms of violence highlights the need for "universal" programs to be offered truly universally. Almost all youth will encounter situations where they are at risk for victimization, perpetration, or both, and ideally, every youth would have the benefits of life skills instruction and exposure to nonviolent social norms. But programs are not equally scalable. Most classroom curricula are much harder to "scale up" to national levels than social marketing campaigns.[1] When we compare prevention programs or components of prevention programs, we need to give more attention to developing readily scalable and adoptable programs. Possibilities for using the internet to prevent violence, although common (such as Itgetsbetter.org) have not been evaluated for risks and benefits.

Assessment

Contrary to some popular conceptions, the key social institutions for individuals and families in need primarily serve an assessment or screening function. For example, many families have open child protective services (CPS) cases for a very short time and up to 80 % of CPS-referred children receive no services (English et al. 2005). Many people who seek psychotherapy attend few sessions, and the modal number of therapy sessions remains one in most populations (Chaffee 2007). Given that people who experience or perpetrate violence often are reluctant to identify violence as their presenting problem (Doss et al. 2004), assessment can be a critical opportunity for raising awareness about the importance that perpetration and victimization play in a host of psychological and physical problems.

How Compartmentalization Affects Assessment

Compartmentalization undermines this opportunity primarily because too many social and human service agencies define their mandate very narrowly to address the referral issue or presenting problem. By limiting assessment to the presenting problem, agencies miss the opportunity to understand and intervene in an array of factors that may be compromising clients' functioning. The true mission of most agencies is

---

[1] We are indebted to Kiersten Stewart of Futures Without Violence for drawing our attention to this issue.

to ensure the welfare of children, families, or the broader population—ranging from schools to child protection services to law enforcement to healthcare. A "bandaid" approach to helping people vulnerable to victimization or changing the behavior of people who commit violence against others falls well short of that mission.

Improving Assessment Through Greater Emphasis on Co-occurrence

The interlinkages among violence types indicate that the goals and tools of assessment need a broader focus. Some existing initiatives have already taken steps in these directions.

First door, right door. The "no wrong door" concept was first introduced for substance abuse treatment (Center for Substance Abuse Treatment 2000). In a no wrong door approach, individuals are assessed and either treated or referred no matter where they first enter the realm of services. The concept recognizes that individuals with multiple problems and needs are likely to enter "the system" at a single entry point, but that this point of first contact may not be the best place to meet their needs. Members of the public may not know which services are best suited to their needs, or they may enter the system involuntarily through law enforcement. Instead of sending people away who have inadvertently found their way to the wrong service agency, the "no wrong door" philosophy promotes the offering of sufficient help with referrals and coordination so that help-seeking in itself is not inadvertently discouraged. "No wrong door" has continued to gain prominence as a way to improve services in many fields, including those with co-occurring substance abuse and mental health disorder (e.g., Sacks and Ries 2005). It is also consistent with the US Department of Justice's Defending Childhood Initiative, which includes a focus on interagency cooperation. Assessments for the co-occurrence of violence would mesh readily with a "no wrong door" philosophy, and could be integrated into the more detailed screenings that are being put into place at many human and social service agencies.

Instruments for assessing multiple forms of violence. The goal of broadly assessing multiple forms of violence requires comprehensive measures that can be readily used in a range of clinical and social service contexts. To be maximally useful, these measures need to be relatively brief, reliable, and valid. Space does not permit a detailed review, but a few examples suggest the range of possibilities. The Juvenile Victimization Questionnaire (Finkelhor et al. 2005) assesses more than 40 types or subtypes of victimization across five general areas: conventional crime, maltreatment, peer and sibling victimization, sexual victimization, and witnessing and indirect exposures to violence. The CDC's new National Intimate and Sexual Violence Survey (Black et al. 2011) assesses multiple types of physical and sexual victimizations among adults. On the perpetrating side, there are a number of widely used measures, particularly of delinquency and youth violence, such as Elliott and colleagues' widely used questionnaire (Elliott et al. 1985).

Next Steps: Advancing Assessment Through Greater Emphasis on Co-occurrence

1. *Make assessment of co-occurrence the norm, not the exception.* Children referred to CPS should also be asked about victimizations in school and the community. Adults mandated to batterers' intervention should be asked about other violence they may have committed as well as about victimization experiences (the latter is especially important for gender-sensitive interventions). Children referred to bullying in the schools should be asked about safety at home. These are all highly overlapping populations, and it will be impossible to create safe families, safe schools, and safe communities without addressing this overlap.

2. *Incorporate the assessment of violence and safety into all clinical contacts.* This could be done similarly to screens for suicidal or homicidal ideation. Typically, regardless of the presenting problem, brief screens regarding suicidal or homicidal ideation are automatically included in virtually every clinical intake or crisis intervention. Even a one-sentence screen, such as "Have you been hurt by someone in the last year, or do you ever feel scared or unsafe at home, school, or in your neighborhood?" could improve identification. The Affordable Care Act now requires that screening and counseling for interpersonal and domestic violence are offered as no-cost-sharing preventive care for women, and this could be extended to men and youth.

3. *Explicitly address the needs of all family members.* Too many services focus on a single family member, rather than the whole family, as "the" client. In particular, the needs of victimized parents should be more formally incorporated into child protection assessments. A parent's ability to implement CPS recommendations will depend in part on her ability to freely choose her actions, and if she is also a victim, this may not be the case. At least anecdotally, many child protection assessments of parents are still very adversarial (Sirotkin and Fecko 2008), and it is unlikely that an adversarial approach serves the long-term interests of families.

Similarly, the high degree of co-occurrence among forms of family violence indicates that screening for child victimization in domestic violence agencies should be more widely implemented. Dangerousness assessments and safety planning could explicitly incorporate risks to children to help parents develop plans that respond to those risks. An instrument such as the VIGOR (Victim Inventory of Goals, Options, and Risks) is one possible tool (Hamby and Clark 2011). Many shelters house almost as many children as adults (for example, 47 % of shelter residents are children in North Carolina, North Carolina Council for Women 2009), and children should not actually reside in a social service program without having their needs assessed.

Evaluate the merits of different approaches to screening and assessment. More research needs to be done to establish the best assessment approaches. As with prevention programs, research should include head-to-head comparisons of assessments, not just determine whether assessments or screens are better than their absence. More research also needs to be done to determine how to make assessment and screening functions most helpful for people who do not receive further services. For example, DeBoer et al. (2012) recently found that about one-third of couples who were refused conjoint therapy because of intimate partner violence levels that exceeded the criteria for one program simply went and sought couples' therapy elsewhere. Unfortunately, subsequent couples' therapy did not reduce violence incidence for these couples. This suggests preliminary screening and feedback could better steer clients to suitable services.

Intervention

Our recommended strategies for intervention largely parallel those for assessment. The recognition of co-occurrence as the norm, not the exception, should become a central organizing principle when intervening with children, adults, and families. Although few interventions focus specifically on violence co-occurrence, there have been many approaches that have had a wider focus. Thus, it is possible to identify several programs that have elements that might serve as models for a web-informed approach to violence intervention.

How Compartmentalization Affects Intervention

The data on co-occurrence indicate that, contrary to the widespread beliefs of people in any number of silos, there is no such thing as the "most critical trauma" or "most toxic experience". Clinicians who specialize in many areas are used to thinking of their specialty—whether it be child sexual abuse, exposure to domestic violence, or something else—as the cause of all of the symptoms that they are seeing and the organizing event of a victim's life. Some clinicians use emblematic stories of particularly horrific events that fall within their specialty to illustrate this. But the data on co-occurrence suggests that it is repeated victimization, in multiple settings and at the hands of multiple perpetrators, that characterizes the lives of many individuals, especially those most likely to seek help. What kind of trauma is "worst" varies across people and depends on the particular constellation of experiences that individuals have had. As with screening, compartmentalization affects intervention in that far too many services are organized toward treating just a single family member.

Next Steps: Advancing Intervention Through Greater Emphasis on Co-Occurrence

1. *Focus on all family members.* The importance of this principle extends beyond assessment. For example, given the very high percentage of IPV victims who are parents, treatment plans which direct nonoffending parents to immediately leave the perpetrator may not always stop the violence. Frequent mention is made of the risks of separation violence, which is the persistence or initiation of assault

and stalking after separation (e.g., Tjaden and Thoennes 2000). According to some data, the majority of intimate partner femicides occur in couples who have had at least one separation in the past year (Campbell et al. 2007). These risks need to be more thoroughly integrated into treatment plans. A realistic, safe plan would involve careful risk assessment and sufficient offers of resources and support, rather than stronger directives to terminate the parental relationship or lose custody of the children. More cooperative approaches, such as Parent–Child Psychotherapy (Lieberman et al. 2005), show considerable promise and could be implemented more widely. For example, Graham-Bermann et al. (2007, 2011) provide concurrent groups for children exposed to family violence and their mothers that focus on understanding and coping with their violence exposure, and, for mothers, enhancing parenting. In families that participated in both groups, children exhibited larger decreases in internalizing and externalizing behavior problems than in families receiving only the child-focused intervention.

2. *Provide a tighter developmental focus to interventions.* In many respects, a 6-year old who has been abused by a parent has needs that are more similar to a 6-year old who is bullied at school than to a 16-year old abused by a parent. Organizing services by developmental stages, rather than violence types, would be consistent with knowledge about the developmental patterns of violence. For example, bullying peaks in middle childhood, while sexual assault and exposure to community violence accelerate to their highest rates in adolescence and young adulthood. Young parents are most at risk for perpetrating child abuse. Services that offer a "one-size-fits-all" approach to individuals at all developmental stages will be hard-pressed to adequately address the patterns of interrelationships that are distinct to each developmental period. Organizing services by the type of abuse is less child centered than organizing services by child characteristics. Our current organization of services largely emerged through historical accident and need not be reified.

Challenges in Making Assessment and Intervention More Informed by Co-occurrence

1. *Moving from* "trauma-informed care" *to* "victimization-informed care". Trauma-informed care is consistent with the co-occurrence framework because it encourages providers from a wide range of settings to evaluate exposure to violence (Harris and Fallot 2001). One key limitation, however, is that the emphasis on "trauma" puts the focus on manifest distress and admitted fear. Many victims do not show clinically elevated levels of distress. There are social pressures against trauma symptom disclosure for many groups, such as men from most Western cultures. Just because someone does not disclose trauma-related symptoms does not mean that they are unaffected by victimization or currently safe. Exposure to violence itself should be assessed in a victimization-informed approach to care.

2. *Changing institutional culture.* The culture of a given agency, "how we do things around here," embodies the collected wisdom of the agency staff. However,

long-established cultures also can create inertia that makes change difficult as new evidence and insights are accumulated. We know much more about violence, and the interconnections among violence, than we did 20 or even 10 years ago, and incorporating that new knowledge into existing organizational procedures inevitably will involve some growing pains. However, there are models that offer new approaches to working with victims of violence. Movements, such as children's advocacy centers (CACs), are working toward a focus on holistic services that meet the needs of children, families, and adults, rather than on narrower concerns about fulfilling specific mandates or saving costs. There are processes, such as the sanctuary model (Bloom 2010), to facilitate these change processes that hopefully will become more widely adopted.

3. *"Failure to protect"* and *mandatory reporting for exposure to domestic violence*. As we have shown, intimate partner violence and child abuse often co-occur in the same family. This is true not only for physical child abuse, but other forms of maltreatment including neglect, sexual abuse by known adults, and custodial interference (Hamby et al. 2010). Rather than promoting integrated services for families, as we recommend, one unfortunate way that the intersections among types of violence has been dealt with is by use of child protection policies such as "failure to protect." Under the rubric of "failure to protect," a victimized, nonoffending parent (most often the mother) can be substantiated as neglectful because of their victimization. Unfortunately, this approach places the responsibility for ending the violence on the victim instead of the perpetrator.

Failure to protect is a relatively new use of neglect charges. It was essentially unheard of in the 1970s when mandatory reporting was first established. Including "exposure to domestic violence" as a form of maltreatment is also relatively new. As with failure to protect, it is seldom explicitly identified in legislation, but it is now commonly substantiated as either emotional abuse or neglect in many jurisdictions. These forms of co-occurrence certainly should be addressed, but failure to protect charges and child protection intervention for exposure to domestic violence are nonevidence-based practices that have never been evaluated and may have harmful effects, especially if they lead to unnecessary removal of children from their parents or discourage help-seeking by nonoffending parents. We are opposed to this approach with families. Societal institutions should continue to place the responsibility for violence on perpetrators, not victims.

The adverse consequences of many common child protection interventions need much greater consideration. As stated earlier, simply separating the parents does not always end the violence (Tjaden and Thoennes 2000), but the well-documented phenomenon of separation violence has yet to be well recognized in the child protection field. Ordering parents to separate may actually put children at increased risk for some kinds of victimization, including homicide. Removing children from their parents is also traumatic to children and should only be used as a last resort. The current foster care system also has well-known limitations in terms of imperfect vetting of families. There is no evidence suggesting that witnessing violence warrants extreme interventions.

Instead, we recommend a more holistic, family-centered approach to investigations for family violence. There have been efforts to craft model policies that specifically address exposure to domestic violence and cases of multiple victims in one family, perhaps most notably the Greenbook (Schechter and Edleson 1999). The Greenbook, which provides guidance for judges in family court, recommends that, especially in cases of low or moderate severity, children be kept with nonoffending parents and services be made available without the necessity of opening a child protection investigation. Less coercive approaches are common in many jurisdictions. Although most people practicing in the US today probably cannot remember a time when mandatory reporting did not seem a basic and automatic way of handling child abuse, it is far from a global practice. Many countries, including other wealthy, industrialized stable democracies such as Germany, the United Kingdom, and New Zealand (Mathews and Kenny 2008), use some version of a voluntary reporting system for dealing with cases of child maltreatment. Further, mandatory reporting was implemented well before the importance of evidence-based practice was widely recognized, and the merits of different variations of mandatory reporting policies would be worth investigating in formal program evaluations. Common child protection interventions, such as foster placement and court interventions, are not the solution for reducing violence against children. In recent years, however, there is a growing evidence base for the kinds of programs that do help children in violent families, such as early home visitation which prevents considerable amounts of maltreatment (Olds 2006).

Existing Efforts to Improve Intervention Through Greater Emphasis on Co-Occurrence

Several existing interventions either implicitly or explicitly adopt a co-occurrence philosophy. Although not intended to be an exhaustive list, we offer a few illustrations of services or program philosophies that best exemplify the comprehensive, holistic approaches that seem best suited to addressing the extensive interconnections among forms of violence. None of these offer quick or guaranteed solutions to the problem of violence; indeed, it is unlikely that any such easy solution exists. Further, we are also aware that not every local incarnation of these models lives up to the aspirational goals of their designers (Durlak and DuPre 2008). Nonetheless, in contrast to more piecemeal approaches or more narrowly focused programs, these programs offer ideas about how to develop more effective efforts to minimize all forms of violence. It seems likely that more effective strategies might be based on more strategically coordinated combinations of several of the programs and/or program philosophies described here.

Zero to Three. One of the most important features of the Zero to Three program (National Center for Infants Toddlers and Families 2011), and those like it, is its focus on a specific developmental period. The mission of the program is to ensure that all children are provided the opportunities and resources to successfully master the developmental milestones of this period. Although preventing maltreatment is one of the major goals of Zero to Three, the organization recognizes that this is best accomplished by attending to the full context of the child and family. Zero to Three does this by promoting well-child care, good developmental monitoring, early screening for a wide range of behavioral and mental problems, parental education, child-friendly policies, and other activities to promote the total well being of infants and toddlers. Early nutrition, adequate verbal interaction with parents, and a host of other environmental factors play major roles in neurologic development during these years. Successful passage through this developmental period leaves children physically and emotionally capable of facing later developmental challenges and adversities.

Big Brother, Big Sister, and other mentoring programs. Big Brother/Big Sister (BBBS) is perhaps one of the oldest models to formally adopt a holistic approach. It is still one of the best-known models among the general public, and it shares many elements with the home visitation programs and other new incarnations of intensive, home-centered approaches. The first formal evaluations of BBBS, using a wait-list control group compared to those matched with a BBBS, found that youth in BBBS were approximately one-third less likely to hit someone. A number of other key risk factors, such as drug use initiation, were also reduced (Tierney and Grossman 1995). Since that first large-scale study, the effects of mentoring programs have been much debated. Current evidence suggests most mentoring programs have small to moderate positive effects (Rhodes 2008). Outcomes appear to depend very much on the dosage (frequency and length of contact) and quality of the mentoring relationship. Low-quality mentoring relationships of short duration may even have adverse effects. Nonetheless, with appropriate screening, structure, and supervision, existing data suggest that mentoring has a positive impact on delinquent behaviors and other important youth risk factors, which is particularly noteworthy considering that many programs primarily comprise volunteers working through nonprofit agencies. Unlike the mandates (real or implied) under which many child protection caseworkers, pediatricians, teachers, or prevention providers operate under, most mentors are specifically encouraged to focus on the whole person (Tierney and Grossman 1995). No topic is considered outside the realm of the relationship.

Natural helpers. "Natural helpers" are those who seem able, without formal professional training in therapy techniques, to make a positive impact on other people's lives. They might be coaches, ministers, scout leaders, or teachers. They might be volunteer sponsors in Alcoholics Anonymous or parole officers. They might be grandparents or other members of an extended family. They could be a supportive intimate partner. Although similar to mentors in many ways, natural helpers provide even less formally organized interventions, and researching their impact is challenging. We acknowledge that many of the effective elements of these relationships may be lost were they to become institutionalized. Nonetheless, we think it is important that, retrospectively, many adults identify natural helpers as key to their resilience and survivor (Waller and Patterson 2002). Natural helpers provide another exemplar of a more holistic approach to help. They also serve important and still under-recognized roles, because many people exposed to violence or engaged in the perpetration of violence will not seek help from formal agencies.

Community-Level Interventions: Policy, Law, and Community Action

How Compartmentalization Affects Community-Level Interventions

As already suggested by much of the foregoing, compartmentalization is also seen at the community and even societal levels. Compartmentalization has broad impacts on the ways that policies are developed and implemented, including the development and implementation of laws regarding violence. It also affects community organizing. Perhaps the key impact is on the unintentional overlap and even competition that is created across and even within organizations due to the ad hoc ways that institutional responsibilities are developed. The founding of institutions themselves sometimes is done in an ad hoc manner, often as a reaction to a crisis rather than a planful part of a coherent agenda. Compartmentalization is also seen over time, but many problems are treated as if they are stand-alone incidents instead of part of a general pattern. This is particularly true of law enforcement and healthcare, which are oriented toward treating violence as a one-time emergency, but can be seen in many organizations.

Improving Community Approaches Through Greater Emphasis on Co-occurrence

Coordinated community responses. Many people have called for a more coordinated and integrated approach to institutional organization, such as the meta-leadership model (Marcus et al. 2006). The idea behind meta-leadership and similar initiatives is to make certain that broader societal goals are not forgotten as agencies pursue their own self-interests in addition to the stated mission of their organization. Although they do not typically go by the "meta-leadership" name, there have been a large number of such initiatives in the violence community, including CACs developed to address child sexual abuse and other forms of maltreatment (Walsh et al. 2007), coordinated community response teams for domestic violence (Shepard and Pence 1999), sexual assault response teams, and fatality review teams for both child abuse and domestic violence. Although less common than these other initiatives, the model has also been extended to elder abuse (McNamee and Mulford 2007).

More coordinated approaches offer many potential benefits for public institutions such as law enforcement and child protection and even for some private organizations that provide important public services, such as hospitals and domestic violence shelters. These coordination efforts unfortunately have received little formal study, but there is some evidence in support of them. For example, children seen at CACs for child sexual abuse are more than twice as likely as other victims to receive a formal forensic interview (Walsh et al. 2007), and arrests are more likely when victims are served by sexual assault response teams than by traditional services (Nugent-Borakove et al. 2006). As these findings suggest, greater involvement of law enforcement has often been a key goal of these efforts.

The benefits of coordination may vary for different types of agencies. For many grassroots organizations that focus on raising awareness, social marketing, or developing new programs, some balance between coordination and maintaining independence is probably warranted. An overly centralized focus is antithetical to what is meant by grassroots organizing, but greater communication and resource sharing could help many nonprofits, most of which operate on shoestring budgets.

Legal changes. Another important societal-level approach is legal reform. In the last 100 years or so, with an acceleration over the last 30 or 40 years in many societies, new or revised laws have redefined what is considered violence in the eyes of the law. Most of these efforts have expanded the focus of the criminal justice system, by explicitly labeling child abuse, intimate partner violence, marital rape, and related offenses as criminal. In the US, perhaps the latest legal trend is increasing school responsibilities for the oversight of peer bullying.

Next Steps: Advancing Community Approaches Through Explicit Emphasis on Co-occurrence

1. *Coordinate across silos, not just within them.* Most coordination efforts, despite their sometimes more inclusive-sounding names, are focused on a single form of violence such as child sexual abuse or intimate partner violence. The result is that, especially in larger or wealthier communities, there may be multiple "coordination" efforts going at the same time. An institution or organization that serves victims of many types of violence, such as a hospital or law enforcement, may sit on several such coordinating committees, in some cases even with the same people from other agencies. Yet, the work is still essentially very siloed. Attention may be drawn to the fact that the mother of the child discussed at the CAC is also a client involved with the coordinated response for domestic violence but usually there is no systematic attempt to do so. These coordination efforts could be much more person-centered and family-centered rather than organized around specific types of violence.

2. *Move away from an incident-based approach.* As identified in Chap. 2, patterns across time are just as important as interconnections across diverse forms of violence, but law enforcement and healthcare are organized to treat each act of violence and each traumatic injury as a one-time emergency, an act of

mono-perpetration. Aside from giving stricter sentences to polyperpetrators with prior convictions, there are very few elements in either of these systems to deal with individuals who are entangled in multiple types of violence. This is especially a disservice to victims, whose enduring vulnerabilities may remain long after the arrest or the treatment of any specific injury. The burdens on both of these systems could be reduced if polyperpetrators and polyvictims were identified earlier and tracked into alternative interventions sooner than those for whom violence is truly a monoincident, such as the randomly chosen victim of a mugging who is not usually at high risk for violence.

3. *Explore further uses of social marketing.* In recent years, there has been a more intentional effort to transform the public service announcements of old into more sophisticated public health campaigns that make use of the skills and research developed in the marketing profession. Marketers are very good at selling all kinds of commodities and some advocates are starting to research how the principles of nonviolence and egalitarianism can be "sold" to the general public as a means of shifting social norms in a less violence-approving direction (e.g., Potter et al. 2011). At the time of this writing, these campaigns are just beginning to be subjected to formal program evaluations, although Potter and colleagues did find some increases in intention to intervene in their project. Because social marketing campaigns are much less expensive to run than classroom-based or family-based programs, this is an avenue worth pursuing in future research.

Challenges in Making Community-Level Approaches More Informed by Co-occurrence

1. *Turf wars.* One outcome of the compartmentalization of institutions is that the staff at any institution are vulnerable to adopting a bureaucratic, self-protective, and insular attitude toward their mission that can harm their ability to respond to violence in a way that maximizes outcomes for victims and providers (Marcus et al. 2006). This happens at both governmental and nongovernmental levels, where the basic problems of lack of interagency communication and presence of interagency competitiveness are common. This affects nonprofits (aka nongovernmental organizations) as well, who can jealously guard access to both funding sources and clients if they feel, correctly or not, that sharing information or resources might threaten their viability as an agency. Although we do not envision an easy fix for these issues, more explicit attention to the interests of various stakeholders may help clarify the best approaches to coordination.

2. *Unintended consequences.* The politics of responding to violence can have unintended consequences. The entire field of violence intervention, and most other human services, has become increasingly focused on evidence-based services. Although there can be challenges in documenting the benefits of some services, in general this increasing rigor has been a benefit. To date, however, almost all of the focus on evidence-based services has been focused on programs delivered to individuals or families. As a result, sometimes sweeping organizational and systemic

changes are made without any preliminary evidence supporting whether this is a good idea and with little to no effort to evaluate the outcome of these changes. As described in more detail earlier in the chapter, mandatory reporting and the expansion of mandatory reporting to incidents such as intimate partner violence and elder abuse is one such large-scale change with little to no outcome data. Mandatory arrest for intimate partner violence was implemented in all 50 states and still has only limited and mixed findings in support of it (Sherman 1992). A more evidence-based approach to policy is needed as well.

3. *Coordinating without downsizing.* In today's economic climate, "integration" and "coordination" are often euphemisms for "downsizing" and "reducing services." This is not what we mean by coordination. On the contrary, we are mindful that data continue to show that the main problem with services is underserving people with substantial mental health and behavioral issues (Kazdin and Blase 2011). The emerging recognition of polyvictimization, polyperpetration, and other interconnections is further evidence that many people have needs that are not being sufficiently addressed in the current system, because so many people are receiving services with a very narrow focus on the presenting problem (whether violence or something else such as depression) when they are enmeshed in violence in multiple ways. As has been documented in numerous studies, the majority of individuals who perpetrate or sustain violence receive no services at all. The best hope for increasing our success at reducing violence is not fewer services, but better services with a more coherent organization and delivery system.

Conclusion

New directions are needed to make prevention and interventions of all kinds more effective. Although we have pointed to many types of evidence that are urgently needed to make more informed programing decisions, we are also underutilizing much of the data that we already have. Taking advantage of data on co-occurrence to craft more coordinated, person-centered services has the potential to advance the field and reduce the burden of violence on individuals and families everywhere. Although some of the suggestions we have made would entail fairly large system reform, others can be done simply by broadening the focus of existing services and by taking a more intentional approach to addressing multiple forms of violence.

References

Anderson, L., & Whiston, S. (2005). Sexual assault education programs: A meta-analytic examination of their effectiveness. *Psychology of Women Quarterly, 29*, 374–388.

Ball, B., Kerig, P. K., & Rosenbluth, B. (2009). "Like a family but better because you can actually trust each other": The expect respect dating violence prevention program for at-risk youth. *Health Promotion Practice, 10*, 45S–58S.

Banyard, V. (2011). Who will help prevent sexual violence: Creating an ecological model of bystander intervention. *Psychology of Violence, 1*(3), 216–229.

Black, M., Basile, K., Breiding, M., Smith, S., Walters, M., Merrick, M., et al. (2011). *The national intimate and sexual violence survey: 2010 summary report.* Atlanta: Centers for Disease Control and Prevention.

Bloom, S. (2010). Organizational stress as a barrier to trauma-informed service delivery. In M. Becker & B. Levin (Eds.), *A public health perspective of women's mental health* (pp. 295–311). New York: Spring.

Campbell, J. C., Glass, N., Sharps, P., Laughon, K., & Bloom, T. (2007). Intimate partner homicide: Review and implications for research and policy. *Trauma, Violence and Abuse, 8*(3), 246–269.

Center for Substance Abuse Treatment. (2000). *Improving substance abuse treatment: The national treatment plan initiative.* Washington: U.S. Department of Health and Human Services.

Chaffee, R. B. (2007). Managed care and termination. In W. T. O'Donohue & M. Cucciare (Eds.), *Terminating psychotherapy: A clinician's guide* (pp. 3–14). New York: Routledge.

Chandrasekaran, C., & Hamby, S. (2010). *Lifetime exposure to violence prevention programs in a college sample. Paper presented at the International Family Violence & Child Victimization Research Conference.* Portsmouth, NH.

Connell, A. T. D., Yasui, M., & Kavanagh, K. (2007). An adaptive approach to family intervention: Linking engagement in family-centered intervention to reductions in adolescent problem behavior. *Journal of Consulting and Clinical Psychology, 75*, 568–579.

Coté, S., Vaillancourt, T., LeBlanc, J., Nagin, D., & Tremblay, R. (2006). The development of physical aggression from toddlerhood to pre-adolescence: A nationwide longitudinal study of Canadian children. *Journal of Abnormal Child Psychology, 34*, 71–85.

De Bellis, M. (2001). Developmental traumatology: The psychobiological development of maltreated children and its implications for research, treatment, and policy. *Development and Psychopathology, 13*, 537–561.

DeBoer, K., Rowe, L., Frousakis, N., Dimidjian, S., & Christensen, A. (2012). Couples excluded from a therapy trial due to intimate partner violence: Subsequent treatment-seeking and occurrence of IPV. *Psychology of Violence 2*(1), 28–39.

Dishion, T., & Stormshak, E. (2007). *Intervening in children's lives: An ecological, family-centered approach to mental health care.* Washington: American Psychological Association.

Doss, B., Simpson, L., & Christensen, A. (2004). Why do couples seek marital therapy? *Professional Psychology: Research and Practice, 35*, 608–614.

Durlak, J. A., & DuPre, E. P. (2008). Implementation matters: A review of research on the influence of implementation on program outcomes and the factors affecting implementation. *American Journal of Community Psychology, 41*, 327–350.

Elliott, D. S., Huizinga, D., & Ageton, S. S. (1985). *Explaining delinquency and drug use.* Beverly Hills: Sage.

English, D. J., Edleson, J. L., & Herrick, M. E. (2005). Domestic violence in one state's child protective caseload: A study of differential case dispositions and outcomes. *Children and Youth Services Review, 27*, 1183–1201.

Finkelhor, D., Turner, H., Ormrod, R., & Hamby, S. L. (2005). The victimization of children and youth: A comprehensive, national survey. *Child Maltreatment, 10*(1), 5–25.

Finkelhor, D., Ormrod, R., Turner, H., & Holt, M. (2009). Pathways to poly-victimization. *Child Maltreatment, 14*(4), 316–329.

Foshee, V., Linder, G., Bauman, K., Langwick, S., Arriaga, X., Heath, J., et al. (1996). The safe dates project: Theoretical basis, evaluation design, and selected baseline findings. *American Journal of Preventive Medicine, 12*, 39–47.

Foshee, V., Bauman, K. E., Greene, W. F., Koch, G. G., Linder, G. F., & MacDougall, J. E. (2000). The safe dates program: 1-year follow-up results. *American Journal of Public Health, 90*, 1619–1622.

Foshee, V., Bauman, K., Ennett, S., Suchindran, C., Benefield, T., & Linder, G. (2005). Assessing the effects of the dating violence prevention program "safe dates" using random coefficient regression modeling. *Prevention Science, 6*, 245–258.

Graham-Bermann, S., Lynch, S., Banyard, V., DeVoe, E. R., & Halabu, H. (2007). Community-based intervention for children exposed to intimate partner violence: An efficacy trial. *Journal of Consulting and Clinical Psychology, 75*(2), 199–209.

Graham-Bermann, S., Sularz, A., & Howell, K. (2011). Additional adverse events among women exposed to intimate partner violence: Frequency and impact. *Psychology of Violence, 1*(2), 136–149.

Hamby, S., & Clark, S. (2011). *Beyond rope ladders & padlocks: A new approach to safety planning*. Paper presented at the Ending Domestic & Sexual Violence: Innovations in Practice & Research Conference, Portsmouth, NH.

Hamby, S., Finkelhor, D., Turner, H., & Ormrod, R. (2010). The overlap of witnessing partner violence with child maltreatment and other victimizations in a nationally representative survey of youth. *Child Abuse and Neglect, 34*, 734–741.

Harris, M., & Fallot, R. (2001). *Using trauma theory to design service systems*. San Francisco: Jossey-Bass.

Jaffe, P. G., Sudermann, M., Reitzel, D., & Killip, S. M. (1992). An evaluation of a secondary school primary prevention program on violence in intimate relationships. *Violence and Victims, 7*(2), 129–146.

Kazdin, A. E., & Blase, S. (2011). Rebooting psychotherapy research and practice to reduce the burden of mental illness. *Perspectives on Psychological Science, 6*, 21–37.

Lieberman, A. F., Van Horn, P., & Ippen, C. G. (2005). Toward evidence-based treatment: Child-parent psychotherapy with preschoolers exposed to marital violence. *Journal of the American Academy of Child and Adolescent Psychiatry, 44*(12), 1241–1248.

Marcus, L. J., Dorn, B. C., & Henderson, J. M. (2006). Meta-leadership and national emergency preparedness: A model to build government connectivity. *Biosecurity and Bioterrorism: Biodefense Strategy. Practice, and Science, 4*(2), 128–134. doi:10.1089/bsp.2006.4.128.

Mathews, B., & Kenny, M. C. (2008). Mandatory reporting legislation in the United States, Canada, and Australia: A cross-jurisdictional review of key features, differences, and issues. *Child Maltreatment, 13*(1), 50–63. doi:10.1177/1077559507310613.

McNamee, C., & Mulford, C. (2007). *Innovations assessment of the elder abuse forensic center of orange county, California (NCJ 220331)*. Washington: National Institutes of Justice.

Nation, M., Crusto, C., Wandersman, A., Kumpfer, K., Seybolt, D., Morissey-Kane, E., et al. (2003). What works in prevention: Principles of effective prevention programs. *American Psychologist, 58*(6/7), 449–456.

National Center for Infants Toddlers & Families (2011). Zero to Three Retrieved December 20, 2011, from http://www.zerotothree.org/.

Noll, J. G., & Grych, J. H. (2011). Read-react-respond: An integrative model for understanding sexual revictimization. *Psychology of Violence, 1*(3), 202–215.

North Carolina Council for Women (2009). Statistical Bulletin 2007–2008 Retrieved from http://www.doa.state.nc.us/cfw/stats.htm.

Nugent-Borakove, M. E., Fanflik, P., Troutman, D., Johnson, N., Burgess, A., & O'Connor, A. (2006). *Testing the efficacy of SANE/SART programs: Do they make a difference in sexual assault arrest & prosecution outcomes? (NCJRS No. 214252)*. Washington: National Institutes of Justice.

Olds, D. (2006). The nurse–family partnership: An evidence-based preventive intervention. *Infant Mental Health Journal, 27*, 5–25.

Potter, S. (2012). Using a multi-media social marketing campaign to increase active bystanders on the college campus *Journal of American College Health., 60*(4), 282–295.

Potter, S., Moynihan, M. M., & Stapleton, J. G. (2011). Using social self-identification in social marketing materials aimed at reducing violence against women on campus. *Journal of Interpersonal Violence, 26*(5), 971–990. doi:10.1177/0886260510365870.

Repetti, R., Robles, T., & Reynolds, B. (2011). Allostatic processes in the family. *Development and Psychopathology, 23*, 921–938.

Rhodes, J. E. (2008). Improving youth mentoring programs through research-based practice. *American Journal of Community Psychology, 41*, 35–42.

Sacks, S., & Ries, R. (2005). *Substance abuse treatment for persons with co-occurring disorders (SMA 05–3922)*. Rockville: Substance Abuse and Mental Health Services Administration.

Schechter, S., & Edleson, J. L. (1999). *Effective intervention in domestic violence and child maltreatment: Guidelines for policy and practice Reno*. NV: National Council of Juvenile and Family Court Judges.

Shepard, M. F., & Pence, E. L. (Eds.). (1999). *Coordinating community responses to domestic violence: Lessons from duluth and beyond*. Thousand Oaks: Sage.

Sherman, L. (1992). *Policing domestic violence*. New York: Free Press.

Sirotkin, J. N., & Fecko, C. M. (2008). A case study in post-Nicholson litigation. *American Bar Association Commission on Domestic Violence Newsletter, 12*, .

Stormshak, E., & Dishion, T. (2009). A school-based, family-centered intervention to prevent substance use: The family check-up. *The American Journal of Drug and Alcohol Abuse, 35*, 227–232.

Taylor, B., Stein, N., Woods, D., & Mumford, E. (2011). *Shifting boundaries: Final report on an experimental evaluation of a youth dating violence prevention program in New York city middle schools (No 236175)*. Washington: U.S. Department of Justice.

Thornton, T., Craft, C., Dahlberg, L., Lynch, B., & Baer, K. (2002). *Best practices of youth violence prevention: a sourcebook for community action (revised)*. Atlanta: Centers for Disease Control and Prevention.

Tierney, J. P., & Grossman, J. B. (1995). *Making a difference: An impact study of big brothers, big sisters*. Philadelphia: Public/Private Ventures.

Tjaden, P., & Thoennes, N. (2000). *Extent, nature, and consequences of intimate partner violence: Findings from the national violence against women survey*. Washington: National Institutes of Justice.

Tjaden, P., & Thoennes, N. (2006). *Extent, nature, and consequences of rape victimization: Findings from the national violence against women survey*. Washington: National Institutes of Justice.

Waller, M., & Patterson, S. (2002). Natural helping and resilience in a Diné (Navajo) community. *Families in Society, 83*(1), 73–84.

Walsh, W. A., Cross, T. P., Jones, L. M., Simone, M., & Kolko, D. J. (2007). Which sexual abuse victims receive a forensic medical examination?: The impact of children's advocacy centers. *Child Abuse and Neglect, 31*(10), 1053–1068. doi:10.1016/j.chiabu.2007.04.006.

Wolfe, D., Crooks, C., Jaffe, P. G., Chiodo, D., Hughes, R., Ellis, W., et al. (2009). A school-based program to prevent adolescent dating violence. *Archives of Pediatric and Adolescent Medicine, 163*(8), 692–699.

Chapter 7
Conclusion: Toppling the Silos

Recognizing the interrelationships among different forms of victimization and perpetration provides a promising opportunity to develop more powerful theories of interpersonal violence and more effective approaches to prevention and intervention. Considerable, even remarkable, progress has been made in the last 50 years in establishing violence as a major social problem. Many formerly hidden and taboo types of violence, such as child sexual abuse, physical abuse, and intimate partner violence, are now recognized as serious public health problems and not the aberrant behavior of a deviant few. The study of each of these types of violence has led to important insights and interventions that have helped countless adults and children. There are hopeful indicators that several forms of violence are on the decline, as are attitudes endorsing violent solutions to a wide range of stressful interpersonal situations.

Still, as we move forward, new ideas are clearly needed to make continuing progress and to help address some intractable and all-too-common forms of violence. Or perhaps "new" is not the right word. In each silo, over and over again, phenomena such as re-victimization, intergenerational transmission, and perpetrator–victims are "discovered." Some of the findings and models included in this book are years or even decades old. Nonetheless, these findings have not seriously challenged the dominance of the disciplinary silos within which most people work. If we are to fully integrate these data into research and action, doing business-as-usual is an incomplete and insufficient response. Despite the success to date, we are going to be limited in what we can achieve by focusing on different forms of violence in isolation.

Understanding the patterns that connect different forms of abuse, maltreatment, and violence over time and across contexts represents a "second wave" of violence scholarship (Hamby 2011) that has the potential to transform research and intervention in the field. In preceding chapters, we have outlined many specific research, prevention, and intervention implications that are suggested by the impressive degree of interconnection among types of violence. We would like to close by emphasizing four primary themes that can guide this new generation of work on violence.

S. Hamby and J. Grych, *The Web of Violence*, SpringerBriefs in Sociology,
DOI: 10.1007/978-94-007-5596-3_7, © The Author(s) 2013

Extend and Expand Theory and Research

As we discussed in Chap. 5, there are a variety of ways to extend empirical research to incorporate multiple forms of violence. Simply adding one or two closely related forms of violence to a study of another type would contribute to making connections across different silos. More broadly, a co-occurrence framework can guide the development of a comprehensive epidemiology of violence that in turn would inform the development of new theoretical understanding of the resulting patterns. Because the dynamics are similar across types of violence, expanding research does not involve a multifold increase in one's knowledge base, but rather mastering a framework of common and unique risk factors. Although these goals may sound expansive, they will be achieved in a simple way: by individual researchers deciding to broaden the focus of their work to answer new questions.

Integrate and Coordinate Prevention and Intervention Services

Similarly, thinking "outside the silo" by integrating ideas and methods from programs targeting different forms of violence can extend the reach and impact of intervention and prevention efforts. Greater coordination across programs can reduce the duplication and wheel reinvention that consume critical time and resources. For example, individuals interested in creating or evaluating a middle school prevention program do not need to confine the intervention or outcome assessment to a single silo. Rather, thinking developmentally about all of the risks and vulnerabilities those middle schoolers face, or are about to face, and considering how other programs have targeted those factors is likely to have a more powerful impact.

Communicate and Collaborate

Expanding research and intervention to include different forms of violence would be facilitated by increased communication among individuals with different areas of expertise. One of the most expeditious ways to do integrative research is to team up with researchers of different specialties. Organizing symposia at conferences, designing empirical studies, writing papers, and preparing grant applications designed to cut across silos builds on the strengths of the two (or more) investigators and offer opportunities for collaborations that can be innovative, intellectually enriching, and fun.

Incentivize and Institutionalize

Although there are a variety of steps that individuals can take to further understand the interconnections among different forms of violence, the solutions to the problem of compartmentalization do not lie solely in the heroism of researchers and providers taking on new challenges. The way forward will involve changing the systemic incentives that favor or even demand compartmentalization. Encouraging granting agencies, journals, and professional organizations to put more emphasis on co-occurrence in their funding and publication decisions would offer incentives for broadening one's expertise. In grant proposals it could be included as a desirable part of the background, as pilot data are now, or it could also be given more weight in terms of deliverables. An integrative review of a grant's findings, with implications for related fields, could even be made a required deliverable. The addition of a simple criterion to tenure evaluations to document the publication of review, theoretical, meta-analytic, or other synthetic works could change the game considerably in terms of how motivated people are to carve out the time for this more holistic but also labor-intensive scholarship. Journals can highlight research that integrates different forms of violence. For example, the APA journal *Psychology of Violence* has published a special issue on the co-occurrence of violence and explicitly encourages submissions that cut across violence silos (Grych and Swan 2012). Funding opportunities that recognize the value of a broader focus on interpersonal violence could stimulate research and encourage collaboration. In fact, eventually a specific rationale may need to be provided to conduct a study on a single form of violence, and it will be the norm that most professionals will have a good working knowledge of the basic dynamics and consequences for many types of violence, not just one or two.

Professional organizations and agencies could promote cross-training as well. For example, state licensing agencies could incentivize the process by including requirements for continuing education that include training in multiple forms of violence. Agencies such as the Centers for Disease Control and Department of Justice could include similar requirements in service-oriented grants. There also are good models of coordinated community responses, such as Children's Advocacy Centers for child maltreatment (CACs) and Sexual Assault Response Teams (SARTs) for sexual assault. As noted in Chap. 6, there is room for even these models to extend further across silos. For example, CACs could do more to address clients' relationships with peers as well as families.

These are just a few possibilities. Many of them would, no doubt, be trickier to implement widely or scale up than they are to imagine. Nonetheless, breaking down institutional silos can lead to more integrative, comprehensive models of violence, and these types of systemic reforms will be key to developing a more person-centered, less compartmentalized approach to the problem of violence.

Final Thoughts

No form of violence is an isolated phenomenon. As we have shown in the preceding chapters, the interconnections among forms of violence are quite extensive. These interconnections extend across time and across relationships. They affect children, adolescents, and adults. Violence that happens in the home is inextricably linked to violence that happens in communities, schools, and workplaces.

Neighborhoods affect schools and schools affect neighborhoods. These interconnections even extend across roles. Although we cling to the simpler notions of "pure" victims and "pure" perpetrators, the reality is that many individuals are involved in violence as both victim and perpetrator. These interconnections are found in the etiology and developmental pathways that lead to the emergence of violence. Most of the identified causes of violence are general causes that produce many types of violence. They become further enmeshed and intertwined in developmental trajectories that can lead to cascades of escalating risk and vulnerability.

We can turn these interconnections to our advantage as we endeavor to better understand and better respond to the problem of violence. From an intervention perspective, the many interconnections are good news, because they suggest that reductions in one type of violence can radiate outward to produce reductions in other forms of violence. Reducing child abuse, for example, is likely to reduce bullying, teen dating violence, intimate partner violence, and abuse of the next generation of children. The co-occurrence framework offers the hope that the problem is finite. Coordination, integration, and collaboration are the keys to an effective, holistic, person-centered advance toward a violence-free future.

References

Grych, J. H., & Swan, S. (2012). Toward a more comprehensive understanding of interpersonal violence: Introduction to the special issue on interconnections among different types of violence. *Psychology of Violence, 2*(2), 105–110. doi:10.1037/a0027616.

Hamby, S. (2011). The second wave of violence scholarship: Integrating and broadening theories of violence. *Psychology of Violence, 1*(3), 163–165.

CPSIA information can be obtained at www.ICGtesting.com
Printed in the USA
BVOW08s0900040614

355385BV00001B/1/P